Manual for
Eye Examination
and Diagnosis

Eighth Edition

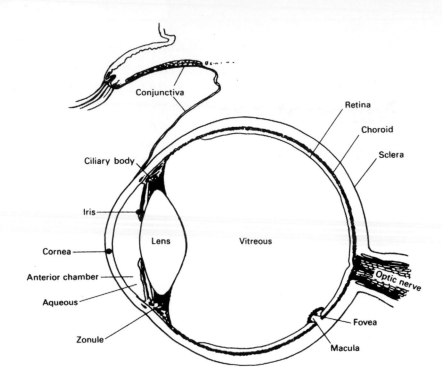

Cornea	Clear, front part of the eye
Iris	Colored diaphragm that regulates amount of light entering
Aqueous	Clear fluid in front part of the eye
Ciliary body	Produces aqueous and focuses lens
Lens	Clear, refracting media that focuses light
Vitreous	Clear jelly filling the back of the eye
Sclera	Rigid, white outer shell of the eye
Conjunctiva	Mucous membrane covering sclera and inner lids
Retina	Inner lining of the eye containing light-sensitive rods and cones
Macula	Avascular area of the retina responsible for the most acute vision
Fovea	A pit in the center of the macula corresponding to central fixation of vision
Choroid	Vascular layer between retina and sclera
Optic nerve	Transmits visual stimuli from retina to brain
Zonule	Fibers suspending lens from ciliary body

Manual for Eye Examination and Diagnosis

Mark W. Leitman MD

Chairman, Department of Ophthalmology
University Surgicenter
East Brunswick
New Jersey, USA

EIGHTH EDITION

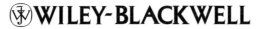

WILEY-BLACKWELL

A John Wiley & Sons, Ltd., Publication

Third Edition 1988
Fourth Edition 1993
Fifth Edition 2001
Sixth Edition 2004
Seventh Edition 2007
Eighth Edition 2012

Library of Congress Cataloging-in-Publication Data
[to come, ISBN 9780470671122]

A catalogue record for this book is available from the British Library.

Set in 8.5 Frutiger Font

Typeset by Aptara Inc. New Delhi, India
Printed and bound in Malaysia by Vivar Printing Sdn Bhd

1 2012

A SERIOUS STUDENT IS LIKE A SEED.

WITH SO MUCH POTENTIAL IT WILL GROW
ALMOST ANYWHERE IT LANDS.

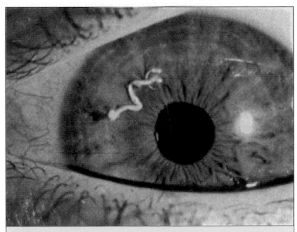

Fig. i A seed introduced into the eye of an 8 year-old boy through a penetrating corneal wound became imbedded in the iris. Many months later, the seed became visible when it began germinating.
Courtesy of Solomon Abel, MD, FRCS, DOMS and *Arch. Ophth.*, Sept. 1979, Vol. 97, p. 1651. Copyright 1979 Amer. Med Assoc.

Contents

Preface

The first edition of this book was started when I was a medical student 40 years ago during the allotted two-week rotation in the eye clinic. At that time, all introductory books were 500 pages or more and could not be read quickly enough to understand what was going on. With this in mind, each word of this 157-page manual was carefully chosen so as to allow the beginning eye care professional to understand the refraction and hundreds of the most commonly encountered eye diseases from the onset. They are discussed with respect to anatomy, instrumentation, differential diagnosis, and treatment in the order in which they would be uncovered during the eye exam, with 534 photos and illustrations.

It is meant to be read in its entirety in a few hours and, hopefully, impart to you a strong foundation on which to grow and enjoy this beautiful and ever-changing speciality. The popularity of previous editions has resulted in translations into Spanish, Japanese, Indonesian, Italian, Russian, Greek, Polish, Portuguese, and an Indian reprint.

My special appreciation goes to Johnson & Johnson's eye care division, which provided a generous grant to distribute the previous edition to 40,000 students. Many of the photographs were generously provided by Pfizer Pharmaceuticals (www.xalatan.com), several journals and many of my friends and colleagues. Elliot Davidoff, who sat next to me in medical school, and is now an assistant Clinical Professor of Ophthalmology at The Ohio State University, surprised me numerous times by sending me images without having to ask.

It is an honor to have been granted permission from so many medical and osteopathic schools to give this 8th edition to 32,000 students. I hope you enjoy reading it half as much as I enjoyed writing it. This manual is unbiased in so far as I have received no monetary funding and I have no association with any company whose products are mentioned in this book.

I would appreciate any recommendations and images which would improve the next edition. You may email me at mark.leitman@aol.com.

MARK W. LEITMAN

Introduction to eye care professionals

As the field of eye care has grown more sophisticated, a team approach by numerous allied health personnel has become essential. Certifying letters after the name indicate the person met minimal entry requirements, and will do continuing education.

Ophthalmologist Training includes four years of college, four years of medical (MD) or osteopathic school (DO) and three years of specialty eye residency training. They may remain a general ophthalmologist, but now more often than not, spend an additional 1–2 years subspecializing in cornea and external disease, vitreoretinal disease, cataracts, glaucoma, neuro-ophthalmology, oculoplastic surgery, pathology, pediatric (strabismus) or uveitis. They often employ three allied health professionals.

Optometrist (OD) After completing four years of college, these doctors attend four years of optometry school. They perform similar tasks as the ophthalmologist. They are only permitted to do laser surgery in one state and they have only some authority to prescribe oral medications in 47 states. They may establish their own practice or work for an ophthalmologist. Subspecialties often include pediatrics and low vision.

Optician (ABO) (American Board of Opticians) These technicians usually do not determine the prescription for eye glasses, but are involved in other aspects of fitting spectacles and contact lenses. They may grind the lenses and put them in frames (laboratory optician) or fit them on the patients (dispensing optician). Their training and certification is highly variable from state to state, but often includes two years at a community college.

Ocularist (BCO, BRDO, FASO) These technicians fit ocular prostheses such as a scleral shell after removal of an eye. After five years of apprenticeship, they are eligible to test for different levels of certification.

Ophthalmic photographers (CRA) These technicians, who do anterior segment and retinal photography, ultrasound, and OCT measurements, may or may not be certified.

Office technicians, with medical supervision, may take histories, measure eye pressure, do refractions and visual fields, maintain instruments, give instruction in contact lens wear, and take visual acuities. They don't have to be certified. If certified, their competence and training are recognized by going from entry level, Certified Ophthalmic Assistant (COA) to Certified Ophthalmic Technician (COT) and then to Certified Medical Ophthalmic Technologist (COMT).

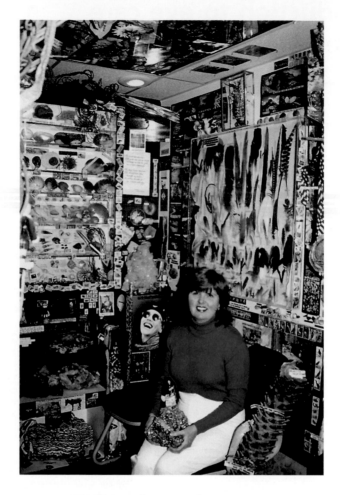

Dedicated to Andrea Kase

It is impossible to perform a good eye exam without a good support team. Andrea has enthusiastically led our team for 31 years as office manager, ophthalmic technician, and typist of all correspondence, including the last six editions of this book. By encouraging me to bring my collection of rocks and other objects from nature into the waiting room, she helped create a museum that my patients look forward to seeing and contributing to.

Chapter 1
Medical history

The history includes the patient's chief complaints, medical illnesses, current medications,
allergies to medications, and family history of
eye disease.

Common chief complaints	Causes
Persistent loss of vision	1 Focusing problems are the most common complaints. Everyone eventually needs glasses to attain perfect vision, and fitting lenses occupies half the eye care professional's day 2 Cataracts are cloudy lenses that occur in everyone in later life. Unoperated cataracts are the leading cause of blindness worldwide. In the USA, over 2.8 million cataract extractions are performed each year 3 Diabetes affects 14 million Americans and is the leading cause of blindness in the USA in those under 65 years of age 4 Macular degeneration causes loss of central vision and is the leading cause of blindness over age 65. Signs are present in 25% of people over age 75 5 Glaucoma is a disease of the optic nerve that Is worsened by elevated eye pressure. It usually occurs after age 35 and affects 2 million Americans, with black persons affected five times as often as white persons. Peripheral vision is lost first, with no symptoms until it is far advanced. Progression to blindness is uncommon if discovered early. This is why there are so many state-sponsored eye-pressure screenings
Transient loss of vision lasting less than $\frac{1}{2}$ hour, with or without flashing lights	In younger patients, think of migrainous spasm of cerebral arteries. With aging, consider emboli from arteriosclerotic plaques
Floaters	Almost everyone will at some time see shifting spots due to suspended particles in the normally clear vitreous. They are usually physiologic, but may result from hemorrhage, retinal detachments, or other serious conditions

Continued on p. 2

Manual for Eye Examination and Diagnosis, Eighth edition. Mark Leitman.
© 2012 John Wiley & Sons, Ltd. Published 2012 by John Wiley & Sons, Ltd.

Common chief complaints	Causes
Flashes of light	Unilateral sparks may be due to traction of the vitreous on the retina which could cause a retinal hole or detachment. Insults to the visual center in the occipital cortex are usually ischemic and cause bilateral jagged lines of light
Night blindness (nyctalopia)	Nyctalopia usually indicates a need for spectacle change, but also commonly occurs with aging and cataracts. Rarer causes include retinitis pigmentosa and vitamin A deficiency
Double vision (diplopia)	Strabismus, which affects 4% of the population, is the condition where the eyes are not looking in the same direction. The binocular diplopia disappears when one eye is covered. In straight-eyed persons, diplopia is caused by hysteria or a beam-splitting opacity in one eye which does not disappear by covering the other eye
Light sensitivity (photophobia)	Usually a normal condition treated with tinted lenses, but could result from inflammation of the eye or brain; internal reflection of light in lightly pigmented or albinotic eyes; or dispersion of light by mucous, lens or corneal opacities, or retinal degeneration
Itching	Most often due to allergy, dry eye, and blepharitis.
Headache	Headache patients present daily to rule out eye causes and to seek direction **1** Headache due to blurred vision or eye-muscle imbalance worsens with use of eyes **2** Tension causes 80–90% of headaches. They typically worsen with anxiety and are often associated with bilateral temple and neck pain **3** Migraine occurs in 18% of women and 6% of men. There is a severe recurrent, unilateral pounding headache often accompanied by nausea, blurred vision, and flashing zigzag lights. It is relieved by sleep **4** Sinusitis causes a dull ache about the eyes and occasional tenderness over the sinus (Fig. 5.3). There may be an associated nasal stuffiness and a history of allergy relieved with decongestants **5** Menstrual headaches are cyclical **6** Sharp ocular pains lasting for seconds are often referred from nerve irritations in the neck, nasal mucosa, or intracranial dura, which like the eye are also innervated by the trigeminal nerve **7** Headaches that awaken the patient and are prolonged or associated with focal neurologic symptoms should be referred for neurologic study
Visual hallucinations	Dementia, psychosis, medications, or reduced sensory stimulation, as in blindness and deafness, especially in the elderly

Medical illnesses

Record all systemic diseases. Diabetes and thyroid disease are two of the most common. Both may be first discovered in an eye examination.

Diabetes mellitus (see cover)

1 Diabetes may be first diagnosed when there are large changes in spectacle correction due to the effect of blood sugar changes on the lens of the eye.
2 Diabetes is one of the common causes of III, IV, and VI cranial nerve paralysis. It is due to closure of small vessels. The resulting diplopia may be the first symptom of diabetes.
3 Cataracts and glaucoma are more common in diabetics.
4 Retinopathy is the most serious complication. If discovered early, laser treatment may reduce visual complications by 50%. Therefore all diabetics should be examined yearly.

Autoimmune (Graves') thyroid disease

This is a condition in which an orbitopathy may be present with hyper- but also hypo- or euthyroid disease.
1 It is the most common cause of bulging eyes, referred to as exophthalmos or proptosis. This is due to fibroblast proliferation and mucopolysacharide infiltration of the orbit. A small white area of sclera appearing between the lid and upper cornea is diagnostic of thyroid disease 90% of the time (Fig. 1.1). This exposed sclera may be a result of exophthalmos or thyroid lid retraction due to an overactive Müller's muscle that elevates the lid. Severe orbitopathy may be treated with steroids, radiation, or surgical decompression of the orbit (Figs 1.2 and 1.3).
2 Infiltration of eye muscles may cause diplopia and is confirmed by a computed tomography (CT) scan (Figs 1.2 and 1.3).
3 Exophthalmos may cause excessive exposure of the eye in the day and an inability to close the lids at night (lagophthalmos), resulting in damage to the cornea.
4 Optic nerve compression could cause permanent loss of vision (Fig. 1.2).

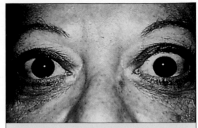

Fig. 1.1 Thyroid exophthalmos with exposed sclera at superior limbus.

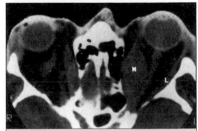

Fig. 1.2 Computed tomography scan of thyroid orbitopathy showing infiltration of medial rectus muscle (M) and normal lateral rectus muscle (L). Compression of left optic nerve could cause optic neuropathy. This is called crowded apex syndrome. Courtesy of Jack Rootman.

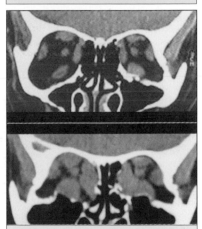

Fig. 1.3 Orbital CAT scan of Graves' orbitopathy before surgical decompression (above) and after right orbital floor osteotomy (below). Often 3, but rarely all 4, bony walls may be opened. Note thickened extraocular muscles. Courtesy of Lelio Baldeschi, MD, and *Ophthalmology*, July 2007, Vol. 114, p. 1395–1402.

Medications

Record patient medications. Below are listed commonly prescribed drugs causing ocular side effects.

Hydroxychloroquine (Plaquenil) is a cornerstone medication used to treat autoimmune diseases, such as rheumatoid arthritis and lupus erythematosus and the parasitic disease malaria. It causes "bulls' eye" maculopathy (Fig. 1.4) and corneal deposits (Fig. 1.12). Long-term use requires the patient to get a baseline exam with an eye doctor before starting medication. It includes at least visual acuity, Amsler grid, color vision, and retina exam to rule out pre-existing maculopathy. The patient should follow-up every six months. Depending on the dosage and the chronicity of use, the eye doctor will determine if additional tests are necessary. Risk increases if dosage exceeds 6.5 mg/kg, especially when taken for more than five years and if there is pre-existing macular degeneration.

The retina is also adversely affected by phenothiazine tranquilizers (Fig. 1.5); niacin, a lipid-lowering agent; tamoxifen, used for breast cancer (Figs 1.7 and 1.8); and interferon used to treat multiple sclerosis and hepatitis C.

Ethambutol, used for tuberculosis, may cause optic neuritis. Corticosteroids may cause cataracts and glaucoma and increase the incidence of herpes keratitis.

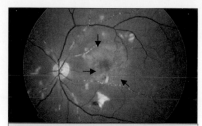

Fig. 1.4 Bull's eye maculopathy due to hydroxychloroquine in patient with systemic lupus. The vasculitis and white cotton-wool spots are due to the lupus. Courtesy of Russel Rand, MD and *Arch. Ophthal.*, Apr 2000, Vol 118, p. 588–589. Copyright 2000, Amer. Med. Assoc. All rights reserved.

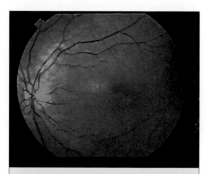

Fig. 1.5 Phenothiazine maculopathy with pigment mottling of macula.

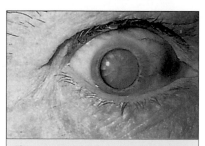

Fig. 1.6 Cataract.

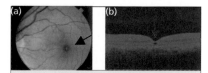

Fig. 1.7 Tamoxifen maculopathy with crystalline deposits (a); and (b) Optical coherence tomography (OCT) showing crystals in the fovea. Courtesy of Joao Liporaci, MD.

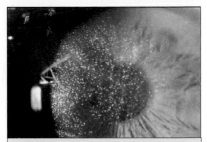

Fig. 1.8 Besides causing maculopathy, tamoxifen also causes crystal deposition in the cornea (keratopathy). Courtesy of Olga Zinchuk, M.D., p. 4 and *Arch. Ophth.*, July 2006, Vol 124, p. 1046.

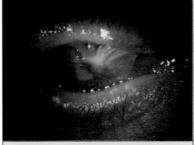

Fig. 1.9 Stevens-Johnson syndrome with inflammation and adhesions of lid and bulbar conjunctiva. Reprinted with permissions from *Amer. J. Opthal.*, Aug 2008, Vol 1 146, p. 271. Surgical strategies for fornix reconstruction. Based on *Symblepharon Severity*, Ahmad Kheirhah, Gabriella Blanco, Victoria Casas, Yasutaka Hayashida, Vadrecu K Raju, Scheffer C. G. Tseng, Copright 2008, Elsevier.

Pilocarpine, used to treat glaucoma, can cause cataracts (Fig. 1.6).

Flomax (tamsulosin), the most common treatment for an enlarged prostate, increases the complications in cataract surgery due to thinning of the iris dilator muscle.

Stevens-Johnson syndrome (Fig. 1.9) is an immunologic reaction to a foreign substance, usually drugs, most commonly sulphonamides, barbiturates, and penicillin. One hundred other medications have also been implicated. It often affects the skin and mucous membranes. It could be fatal in 35% of cases.

Xalatan, Lumigan, and Travatan are the most commonly prescribed glaucoma medications. All three may darken the iris (Figure 1.10) and periorbital skin (eyelids) (Figure 1.11) with lengthening and darkening of the eye-lashes. The side effect of longer, darker lashes has generated a drug, Latisse, which contains the same chemical as Lumigan. It is applied once a day to the upper eyelid lashes for cosmetic reasons.

Amiodarone (Cordarone, Pacerone), one of the most potent antiarrhythmic drugs, and sildenafil (Viagra), tadalafil (Cialis) and vardenafil (Levitra), used to treat erectile dysfunction, have all been suspected of causing nonarteritic anterior ischemic optic

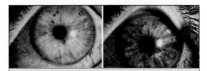

Fig. 1.10 Darkening of a blue iris after 3 months of latanoprost (Xalatan) therapy. This is the most common drug for treating glaucoma. Courtesy of N. Pfelffer, MD and P. Appleton, MD and *Arch. Ophth.*, Feb 2011, Vol 119, p. 191.

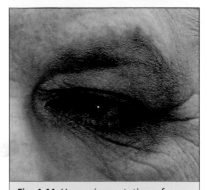

Fig. 1.11 Hyperpigmentation of periorbital skin (eyelids) and iris with darkening and lengthening of lashes.

neuropathy. Amiodarone also causes deposits in the cornea that rarely reduce vision, but may cause glare (Fig. 1.12).

Allergies to medications

Inquire about drug allergies before eye drops are placed or medications prescribed. Neomycin, a popular antibiotic in eye drops, may cause conjunctivitis and reddened skin (Fig. 1.13).

Family history of eye disease

Cataracts, refractive errors, retinal degeneration, and strabismus—to name a few—may all be inherited. In glaucoma, which normally affects 1% of the population, family members have a 10% chance of acquiring the disease. Eighty percent of people with migraine have a relative with the disease.

A special question should be directed to the smoking of cigarettes since it doubles the rate of cataracts, macular degeneration, and all types of uveitis. It also worsens exophthalmos in thyroid disease. Cigarette smoking and smoke-less tobacco use among American adults is about 20%. At age 70, 80% of Americans have high BP and 15% have diabetes. It is predicted that 1 in 3 children born after the year 2000 will develop type II diabetes. One third of Americans are obese and 1/3 are overweight. Remind patients that a major change in lifestyle is needed to stem the pandemic of these chronic diseases. Patients should be reminded about avoiding tobacco and minimizing consumption of red and preserved meats, salt, sugar, and saturated fats. Recommend instead a diet rich in fruits, vegetables, beans, nuts, fish, and whole-grain cereals. Staying thin with a routine daily exercise program should also be advocated.

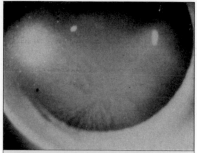

Fig. 1.12 Epithelial deposits radiating from a central point in the inferior cornea. They occur in almost all patients with Fabry's disease, which is an x-linked systemic accumulation of a glycosyphingolipid. Easily seen on slip lamp exam, it can be the first clue in recognizing the presence of this disease which is amenable to therapy. Indistinguishable deposits eventually appear in almost all patients using amiodarone and with hydroxychloroquine. Courtesy of Neal, A., Sher, M.D. and *Arch. Ophth.*, Aug 1979, Vol 97, p. 671–676. Copyright 1979, Amer. Med. Assoc. All rights reserved.

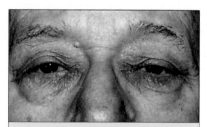

Fig. 1.13 Neomycin allergy occurs in 5–10% of population.

Chapter 2
Measurement of vision and refraction

Visual acuity

The patients read the Snellen chart (Fig. 2.1) from 20 ft with the left eye occluded first. Take the vision in each eye without and then with spectacles.

Vision is expressed in a fraction-like form. The top number is the distance at which the patient reads the chart; the bottom number is the distance at which someone with normal vision reads the same line of the chart. Whenever acuity is less than 20/20, determine the cause for the decreased vision. The most common cause is a refractive error, i.e., the need for lens correction.

If visual acuity is less than 20/20, the patient may be examined with a pinhole. Improvement of vision while looking through a pinhole indicates that spectacles will improve vision. Use an illiterate "E" chart with a young child or an illiterate adult.

Ask the patient which way the ∃ is pointed. Near vision is checked with a reading card held about 14 inches away. If a refraction for new spectacles is necessary, perform it prior to other tests that may disturb the eye.

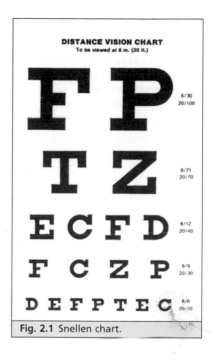

Fig. 2.1 Snellen chart.

Examples of visual acuity	
Measurement in feet (meters in parentheses)	*Meaning*
20/20 (6/6)	Normal. At 20 ft, patient reads a line that a normal eye sees at 20 ft
20/30–2 (6/9–2)	Missed two letters of 20/30 line
20/50 (6/15)	Vision required in at least one eye for driver's license in most states

Continued on page 8

Measurement in feet (meters in parentheses)	Meaning
20/200 (6/60)	Legally blind. At 20 ft, patient reads line that normal eye could see at 200 ft
10/400 (3/120)	If patient cannot read top line at 20 ft, walk him or her to the chart. Record as the "numerator" the distance at which the top line first becomes clear
CF/2ft (counts fingers at 2 ft)	If patient is unable to read top line at 3 ft, have the patient count fingers at maximal distance
HM/3 ft (hand motion at 3 ft)	If at 1 ft patient cannot count fingers, ask him or her direction of hand motion
LP/Proj. (light perception with projection)	Light perception with ability to determine position of the light
NLP	No light perception: totally blind

Record vision as follows			Key	
V $\bar{s}$/	OD	20/70 + 1	V	Vision
	OS	LP/Proj.	$\bar{s}$	Without spectacles
			$\bar{c}$	With spectacles
			OD	Right eye
V $\bar{c}$/	OD	20/20	OS	Left eye
	OS	LP/Proj.	OU	Both eyes

Optics

Emmetropia (no refractive error)

In an emmetropic eye (Fig. 2.2), light from a distance is focused on the retina.

Ametropia

In this disorder, light is not focused on the retina. Four types are hyperopia, myopia, astigmatism, and presbyopia.

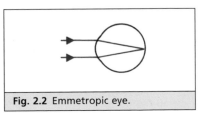

Fig. 2.2 Emmetropic eye.

Hyperopia

Parallel rays of light are focused behind the retina (Fig. 2.3). The patient is farsighted and sees more clearly at a distance than near, but still might require glasses for distance.

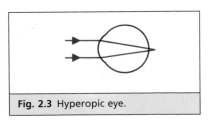

Fig. 2.3 Hyperopic eye.

A convex positive lens is used to correct hyperopia (Fig. 2.4). The power of the lens is expressed in diopters (D). A positive 1 D lens converges parallel rays of light to a focus 1 meter from the lens (Fig. 2.5). The total refracting power of the eye is 60 D; 43 D from the cornea and 17 D from the lens.

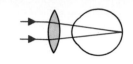

Fig. 2.4 Hyperopic eye corrected with convex lens.

Myopia

Parallel rays are focused in front of the retina (Fig. 2.6). The patient is nearsighted and sees more clearly near than at distance. Myopia often begins in the first decade and progresses until stabilization at the end of the second or third decade. In the past forty years, the prevalence of myopia in young Americans increased from 26% to 43% in whites and 13% to 33% in African-Americans. It has been reported as high as 90% in parts of the Orient. Always strongly linked to inheritance, this new increase is likely due to more near work and less exposure to the outdoors.

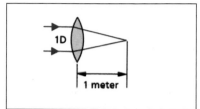

Fig. 2.5 Parallel rays focused by 1 D lens.

A concave negative lens (Fig. 2.7), which diverges light rays, is used to correct this condition.

Refractive myopia is due to increased curvature of the cornea or the human lens, whereas axial myopia is due to elongation of the eye. In axial myopia the retina is sometimes stretched so much that it pulls away from the optic disk (see Fig. 7.6) and may cause retinal thinning (see Fig. 7.7) with subsequent holes or detachments.

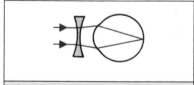

Fig. 2.6 Myopic eye.

Astigmatism

In this condition, which affects 85% of people, the rays entering the eye are not refracted uniformly in all meridians. Regular astigmatism occurs when the corneal curvature is uniformly different in meridians at right angles to each other. It is corrected with spectacles. For example, take the case of astigmatism in the horizontal (180°) meridian (Fig. 2.8). A slit beam of vertical light (AB) is focused on the retina, and (CD) anterior to the retina. To correct this regular

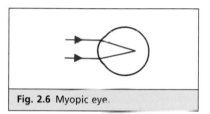

Fig. 2.7 Myopic eye corrected by concave lens.

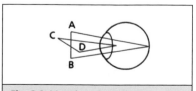

Fig. 2.8 Myopic astigmatism.

astigmatism, a myopic cylindrical lens (Fig. 2.9) is used that diverges only CD.

Irregular astigmatism is caused by a distorted cornea, usually resulting from an injury or a disease called keratoconus (see Figs 6.42 and 6.43).

Presbyopia

This is a decrease in near vision, which occurs in all people at about age 43. The normal eye has to adjust +2.50D to change focus from distance to near. This is called accommodation (see Fig. 6.108). The eye's ability to accommodate decreases from +14D at age 14 to +2D at age 50.

Middle-aged persons are given reading glasses with plus lenses that require updating with age:

40–45 years	+1.00 to +1.50D
50 years	+1.50 to +2.00D
Over 55 years	+2.00 to +2.50D

The additional plus lens in a full reading glass (Fig. 2.10) blurs distance vision. Half glasses (Fig. 2.11) and bifocals (Fig. 2.12) are options that allow for clear distance vision when looking up. No-line bifocals are more attractive, but more expensive.

Refraction

Refraction is the technique of determining the lenses necessary to correct the optical defects of the eye.

Trial case and lenses

The lens case (Fig. 2.13) contains convex and concave spherical and cylindrical lenses and prisms. The diopter power of spherical lenses and the axis of cylindrical lenses are recorded on the lens frames.

Trial frame

The trial frame (Fig. 2.14) holds the trial lenses. Place the strongest spherical lenses in the compartment closest to the eye because

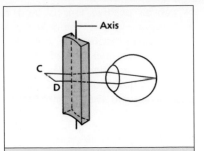

Fig. 2.9 Myopic astigmatism corrected with a myopic cylinder, axis 90°.

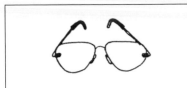

Fig. 2.10 Full reading glass blurs distance vision.

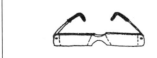

Fig. 2.11 Half glasses.

Fig. 2.12 Bifocals.

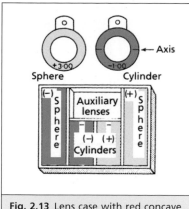

Fig. 2.13 Lens case with red concave and black convex lenses.

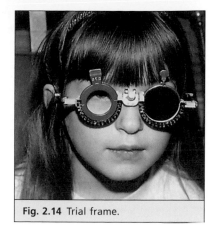

Fig. 2.14 Trial frame.

the effective power of the lens varies with its distance from the eye. Place the cylindrical lenses in the compartment farthest from the eye so that the axis can be measured on the scale of the trial frame (0–180°).

Streak retinoscopy ("flash")

This objective means of determining the refractive error is used to prescribe glasses to infants and illiterate persons who cannot give adequate subjective responses. Hold the retinoscope (Fig. 2.15) at arm's length from the eye and direct its linear beam onto the pupil. To determine the axis of astigmatism, rotate the beam until it parallels the pupillary reflex (Fig. 2.16), then move it back and forth at that axis, as demonstrated in Fig. 2.17.

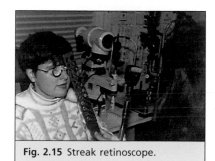

Fig. 2.15 Streak retinoscope.

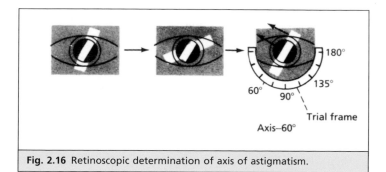

Fig. 2.16 Retinoscopic determination of axis of astigmatism.

If the reflex moves the same way that the retinoscope beam is moving ("with motion"), a plus (+) lens is added to the trial frame. If the reflex moves in the opposite direction ("against motion"), a negative (–) lens is needed. Absence of "with motion" or "against motion" indicates the endpoint. Add –1.50 D to the above findings to approximate the refractive error of that meridian. Rotate the beam 90° to refract the other axis.

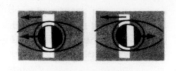

Fig. 2.17 Pupillary reflex with motion and against motion.

Manifest

A manifest is the subjective trial of lenses. Place the approximate lenses, as determined by the old spectacles or retinoscopy, in a trial frame. Occlude one of the patient's eyes, and refine the sphere by the addition of (+) and (–) 0.25 D lenses. Ask which lens makes the letters clearer. Next, refine the cylinder axis by rotating the lens in the direction of clearest vision. Test the cylinder power by adding (+) and (–) cylinders at that axis.

In presbyopes, determine the reading "add" after distance correction.

The following abbreviations are used to record the results of the refraction: W, old spectacle prescription as determined in a lensometer; F, "flash," the refractive error by retinoscopy; M, manifest, the subjective correction by trial and error; Rx, final prescription, usually equal to M.

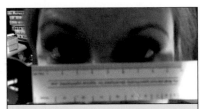

Fig. 2.18 Measurement of interpupillary distance.

A bifocal prescription for a farsighted presbyope with astigmatism is written as shown in Fig. 2.20. The prescription for glasses is determined by an ophthalmologist or an optometrist (OD). That prescription is then given to an optician who fits it into a proper frame. They measure the inter-pupillary distance at near and far (Fig. 2.18) so that the eyes' central visual axis corresponds to the optic centers of the lens. The bifocal height for the particular frame is then measured (Fig. 2.19).

Plastic lenses are typically prescribed because they are lighter and have less chance of shattering. This is especially important in children. Glass has the advantage of being more resistant to scratching.

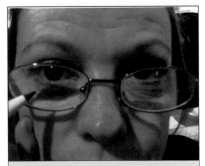

Fig. 2.19 Determination of bifocal segment height.

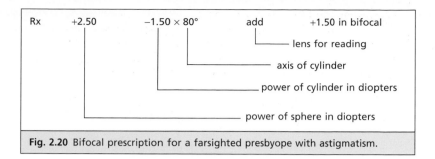

Rx	+2.50	−1.50 × 80°	add	+1.50 in bifocal

— lens for reading

— axis of cylinder

— power of cylinder in diopters

— power of sphere in diopters

Fig. 2.20 Bifocal prescription for a farsighted presbyope with astigmatism.

For photophobia, grey tints are often prescribed because they distort all colors equally. Polaroid lenses minimize glare while driving, boating, or skiing by blocking horizontal light waves. The sun's harmful, ultraviolet UVA and UVB rays may cause skin cancer, photokeratitis, pinuecula (Fig. 6.50) and pterygium (Fig. 6.49a), while hastening the onset of cataracts and macular degeneration. Tinted lenses, including polaroid lenses, should have a UV filter added to remove 98–100% of these rays. Branded photochromic glass lenses and Transitions plastic lenses darken in sunlight and have a UV filter.

Sports injuries, especially basketball, baseball, ice hockey, and racket games, are the leading causes of blindness in children. Protective eye wear could prevent 90% of these sports-related injuries.

Contact lenses

Plastic contact lenses, invented in 1947, are now worn by 34 million Americans, usually as an alternative to spectacles, to correct myopia, hyperopia, astigmatism, and presbyopia (Fig. 2.21).

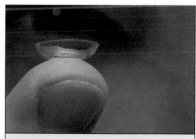

Fig. 2.21 Plastic contact lens.

Other uses of contact lenses include the following:
- Correction of vision in cases of an irregularly shaped cornea
- Tinted and colored lenses for cosmetic effect (see Fig. 2.32) and for reducing photophobia
- Prosthetic artificial eyes to cover a disfigurement or enucleated socket (see Fig. 6.154)
- Bandage lenses relieve discomfort due to blinking associated with corneal abrasions and edema

Candidates for contact lenses

This text will discuss soft lenses since they account for 95% of fittings. Hard and gas-permeable contacts may be preferred less often for cases of dry eye, astigmatism, and irregularly shaped corneas in keratoconus (see Figs 6.42 and 6.43)

Relative contraindications to contact lens wear:

- significant allergies
- lid margin infection
- conjunctivitis
- dry eyes
- very young children or elderly

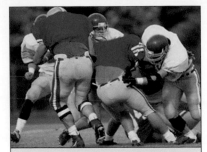

Fig. 2.22 Contacts are great for almost every sport.

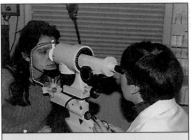

Fig. 2.23 Keratometer.

Fitting contact lenses

Keratometry (Fig. 2.23)

After the refraction for spectacles, the corneal curvature is measured with a keratometer. This determines whether to fit a flatter or steeper lens (see Fig. 2.27). The keratometer also reveals distortion of the cornea from unhealthy contact lens wear (Fig. 2.24) or other corneal diseases.

Power (P), base curvature (BC), and diameter (DIA) are the three basic variables that are usually required to order all types of soft lenses (Fig. 2.25).

Determination of lens power

The power of a contact lens is not always the same as the patient's spectacle correction. Place the contact lens with the spectacle power on the eye. Then, refine it with an over-refraction. The lens should completely cover the cornea and extend just beyond

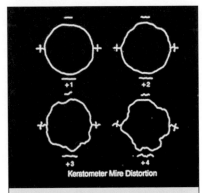

Fig. 2.24 Circular images projected on a damaged cornea have distorted keratometric readings.

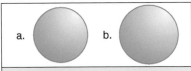

Fig. 2.25 (a) 13.5 mm diameter. (b) 14.5 mm diameter.

the entire limbus (corneal-conjunctival junction) (Fig. 2.26) and move 0.5 to 1.0 mm on each blink. If adequate concentration is not achieved, a different base curve or diameter may be tried.

Types of contact lenses

Most people wear contacts during the day only ("daily wear"). Less often, sleep in lenses ("extended wear") are used, since they have a rate of infection that is 5 times as great as daily wear. Lenses may be replaced yearly, but are more commonly disposed of every 2 weeks to three months ("frequent replacement") or on a daily basis ("disposable"). The frequency of replacement depends on comfort and the rate of mucus accumulation (Fig. 2.28).

Astigmatism lenses are preferred when the astigmatism correction is –0.75 or more. They are elliptical in shape with markings at 90° or 180° axis and weighted at 6 o'clock so they don't rotate (Fig. 2.29). When placed on the eye, these lines should line up close to those axes or an adjustment is made in the axis (Fig. 2.30).

Presbyopic bifocal contact lenses are not highly successful but may be tried for motivated patients—often over age 40—who have problems focusing up close (Fig. 2.31). An alternative to a bifocal contact lens in correcting a presbyopic patient is to use a standard spherical contact lens, making one eye focused for near and the other focused for distance. This is called monovision. Usually, the eye with the clearest vision is chosen for distance.

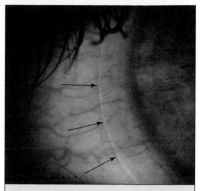

Fig. 2.26 Contact lens properly overlapping limbus.

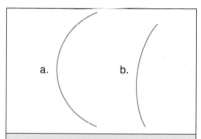

Fig. 2.27 (a) Steep base curve 8.2 mm. (b) Flat base curve 9.1 mm.

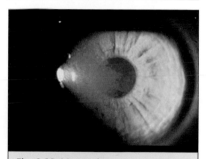

Fig. 2.28 Mucus deposits on contact lenses.

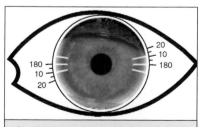

Fig. 2.29 Lens properly aligned on eye with center marking at 180°.

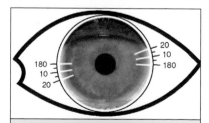

Fig. 2.30 Lens settled on to eye rotated 10° counterclockwise.

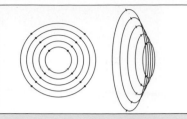

Fig. 2.31 Acuvue bifocal contact lens with concentric zones of alternating near and far vision.

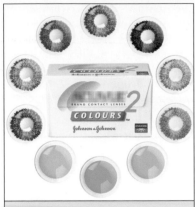

Fig. 2.32 Colored contact lenses.

The iris color could be enhanced with transparent tinted soft lenses or changed to a different color with opaque tinted soft lenses (Fig. 2.32).

No patient should leave the office without feeling adept at lens insertion and removal, realizing the importance of good handwashing techniques, and having knowledge about the use and differences between disinfecting, cleaning, and rinsing (saline) solutions (Figs 2.33–2.35).

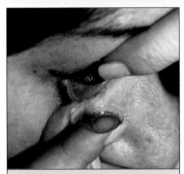

Fig. 2.33 Place contact lens directly on the cornea using the tip of the index finger for the contact, the middle finger to hold lower lid down, and the finger of the other hand to lift upper lid.

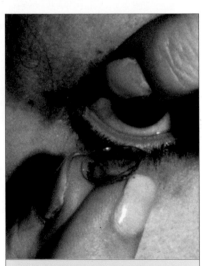

Fig. 2.34 Remove lens by sliding it off cornea onto sclera and then gently pulling it off using thumb and index finger.

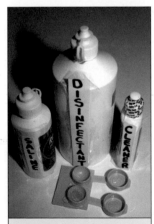

Fig. 2.35 Contact lens solutions.

Common problems

A 2010 study of 144,799 device-associated visits of children to emergency departments showed contact lenses to be the number 1 cause of adverse events (23%). Corneal abrasions, conjunctivitis, and hemorrhage were most frequent.

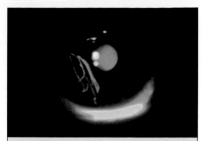
Fig. 2.36 Fluorescein staining of the cornea.

1. Corneal abrasions and edema are highlighted when fluorescein dye is placed in the eye and illuminated with the cobalt blue light. Areas of lost or damaged corneal epithelial cells take up the dye and appear brighter (Fig. 2.36).

2. The upper palpebral conjunctiva is the area most often irritated by contact lenses. Called papillary conjunctivitis (Fig. 2.37), it is often due to contact lens deposits, especially in allergic individuals. it responds well to more frequent replacements.

3. The bulbar conjunctiva surrounding the cornea reddens when the cornea is being compromised as with tight-fitting lenses. (Fig. 2.38).

4. Infected corneal ulcers (Figs 6.21 and 6.22) are the most serious complication and most threatening to vision.

Refractive surgery

The refractive power of the eye may be altered by surgically reshaping the cornea, thereby eliminating the need for distance correction (Fig. 2.39).

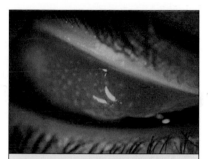
Fig. 2.37 Papillary conjunctivitis with characteristic whitish elevations of conjunctiva.

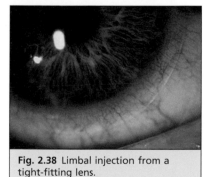
Fig. 2.38 Limbal injection from a tight-fitting lens.

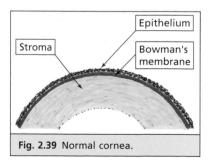
Fig. 2.39 Normal cornea.

Epithelium

Stroma

Bowman's membrane

Refractive surgery began twenty-five years ago in Russia with the radial keratotomy technique (Fig. 2.40). In this procedure, the cornea is flattened with 4–8 radial incisions through 90% of the corneal depth. It has lost popularity due to slow healing, the inability to accurately predict the amount of correction, variable vision throughout the day, glare, halos, infection, and corneal perforation with secondary cataract formation.

Three newer procedures, 1. LASIK, 2. PRK, and 3. epi-LASIK correct myopia, hyperopia, and astigmatism utilizing an excimer laser to remove corneal stroma. In order for the laser to effectively reach the stroma, the corneal epithelium must be gotten out of the way. These three techniques vary in the way this is done.

1. Laser in situ keratomileusis (LASIK—Figs 2.41–2.47) is the most frequently performed elective surgery done in the world with. Many millions have been done since its introduction in 1990. A flap of epithelium, Bowman's membrane, and stroma is created with a blade or femtosecond laser. Then a different laser called an excimer is used to ablate the underlying stromal bed.

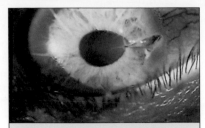

Fig. 2.40 Rare instance of traumatic rupture of radial keratotomy wound. Courtesy of Leo Bores.

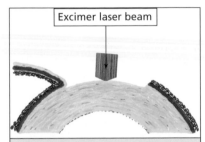

Excimer laser beam

Fig. 2.41 LASIK—Flap of epithelium, Bowman's membrane, and stroma is created with blade or laser. Then, an excimer laser ablates the stroma.

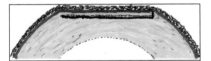

Fig. 2.42 Sculpted cornea after LASIK with remaining Bowman's membrane.

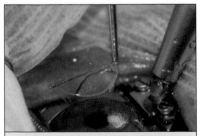

Fig. 2.43 Superficial corneal flap created with microkeratome. Courtesy of Chris Barry, Med Sci, J. Ophthal. *Photography* 1999, Vol 22, No. 1A.

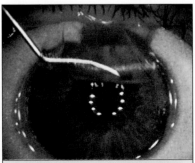

Fig. 2.44 LASIK surgery showing flap being lifted with spatula and laser beam on central cornea ablating stroma. Courtesy of Summit Technology, Inc.

A disadvantage of LASIK is a resulting decrease in ocular rigidity. This is due to loss of ablated stromal bed and decreased effectiveness of stroma remaining in the flap since it never completely heals. To minimize the loss of effective stroma, the goal has been to make the thinnest possible flap. Up to six years later, the flap can still be lifted with a forceps (2.46). In eyes with over 8 diopters of myopia that require a lot of stromal ablation, this combined thinning becomes excessive and could result in an ectasia (bulging) of the cornea. Rarely, it may necessitate a corneal transplant.

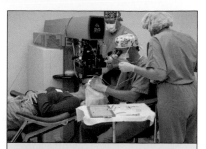

Fig. 2.45 Excimer laser used to remove a layer of central corneal stroma. Courtesy of Summit Technology, Inc.

Because LASIK damages more corneal stroma due to the flap, there is more loss of nerve fibers and a consequential increase in dry eye complaints. Another flap complication is that corneal epithelial cells may grow under the flap and might have to be removed (Fig. 2.47). This occurs in about 1% of primary surgeries, but in up to 23% of cases when the flap has to be lifted for a second LASIK procedure to treat residual refractive error.

2. An alternative to LASIK is photorefractive keratectomy (PRK—Figs 2.48 and 2.49). It avoids creating a flap by mechanically creating a central corneal abrasion. The advantage is it leaves more functioning stroma. The disadvantage is pain from abrasion and slower return of vision.

3. The newest technique, called epi-LASIK (Fig. 2.50) creates an epithelial flap that includes no stroma.

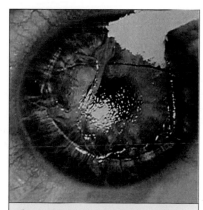

Fig. 2.46 Late dislocation of a LASIK flap by self inflicted injury. Courtesy of C.K. Patel, BSC, FRC Ophth. and *Arch. Ophth.*, Mar. 2001, Vol 119, p. 447. Copyright 2001, Amer. Med. Assoc. All rights reserved.

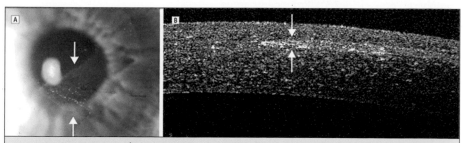

Fig. 2.47 (A) Grey area (↑) where epithelial cells grew under the flap. (B) OCT scan showing cells. If cells are near the central cornea, or if there is overlying melting in the peripheral cornea, the flap must be lifted and cells removed. Courtesy of V. Charistopoulos, MD, and *Arch. Ophth.*, Aug. 2007, Vol. 125, p. 1027–1036. Copyright 2007, Amer. Med. Assoc. All rights reserved.

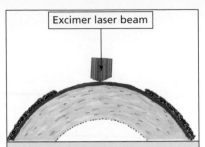

Excimer laser beam

Fig. 2.48 PRK laser ablation of Bowman's membrane and stroma after mechanical debridement of epithelium.

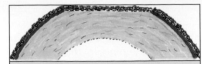

Fig. 2.49 Sculpted cornea after PRK or epi-LASIK.

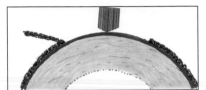

Fig. 2.50 Epi-LASIK. Creation of epithelial flap with blade followed by laser ablation of stroma.

As a consequence there will be more stroma remaining to contribute to ocular rigidity. However, the epithelial flap heals more slowly than the LASIK flap so that vision takes longer to recover. It heals faster and has less pain than PRK where there is a total corneal abrasion after surgery.

All three laser techniques usually yield good results, but may be complicated by infection, glare, halos, dry eye, over- or under-correction of refractive error, and unknown long-term effects. Although LASIK is still by far the most popular technique because of its quick healing, there is a movement toward epi-LASIK because it minimizes dry eye and stromal flap complications.

Intac is a less used technique for correcting small amounts of myopia and keratoconus. It involves the placement of a plastic ring in the peripheral cornea (Fig. 2.51). Proponents argue that unlike LASIK, it is safer because it doesn't involve surgery on the central visual axis.

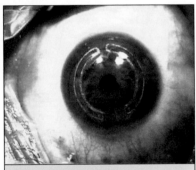

Fig. 2.51 Intac ring. Courtesy of Dimitri Azar, MD.

Large amounts of hyperopia (over 4 diopters) and myopia (over 8 diopters) are difficult to correct with reshaping the cornea because it becomes too thin and unstable. Intraocular lenses can be inserted inside the eye (Fig. 2.52) to correct these larger refractive errors, but have all the inherent risks associated with intraocular surgery. There has to be a safe space between the cornea and the patient's natural lens or corneal edema and/or cataract could occur.

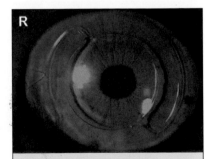

Fig. 2.52 Phakic 6H2 anterior chamber intraocular lens to correct refractive errors. Courtesy of Oii Inc.

Chapter 3
Neuro-ophthalmology

Six muscles move each eye around 3 axes. They are innervated by the III, IV, and VI cranial nerves.

Eye movements

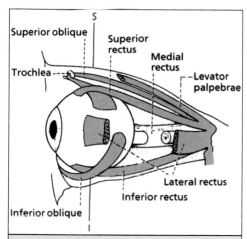

Fig. 3.1 Lateral orbital view: adduction and abduction are around the superior-inferior axis (SI).

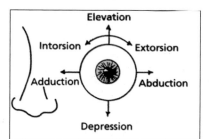

Fig. 3.2 The eye rotates around three different axes coordinated by the action of six extraocular muscles.

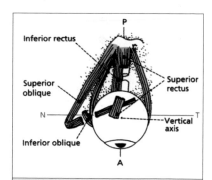

Fig. 3.3 Superior orbital view. Elevation and depression are on the horizontal axis (NT, nasal–temporal) passing from the nasal to temporal side of the eye. Torsion is on the anterior–posterior axis (AP).

Manual for Eye Examination and Diagnosis, Eighth edition. Mark Leitman.
© 2012 John Wiley & Sons, Ltd. Published 2012 by John Wiley & Sons, Ltd.

Six extraocular muscles that rotate the eye

Muscle	Actions	Neural control
Medial rectus	Adducts	Oculomotor nerve (CN III)
Inferior rectus	Mainly depresses, also extorts, adducts	Oculomotor nerve (CN III)
Superior rectus	Mainly elevates, also intorts, adducts	Oculomotor nerve (CN III)
Inferior oblique	Mainly extorts, also elevates, abducts	Oculomotor nerve (CN III)
Superior oblique	Mainly intorts, also depresses, abducts	Trochlear nerve (CN IV)
Lateral rectus	Abducts	Abducens nerve (CN VI)

CN, cranial nerve.

Nerves to ocular structures

	Innervates	Action
Optic nerve Cranial nerve (CN) II	The axon of the retinal ganglion cell which transmits visual impulse from the eye to the brain	
Oculomotor nerve (CN III)		
	1. Medial rectus muscle	Adducts
	2. Inferior rectus muscle	Mainly depresses, also extorts, adducts
	3. Superior rectus muscle	Mainly elevates, also intorts, adducts
Motor (1–5)	4. Inferior oblique muscle	Mainly extorts, also elevates, abducts
	5. Levator palpebrae muscle	Elevates upper lid
Parasympathetic (6–7)	6. Pupil constrictor muscle	Responds to light and near focus
	7. Ciliary muscle	Focuses lens for near
Trochlear nerve (CN IV)	Superior oblique muscle	Mainly intorts, also depresses, abducts
Trigeminal nerve		
	CN V_1 ... Eye, upper lid, orbit, and nose	Sensory
	CN V_2 ... Lower lid	
Abducens nerve (CN VI)	Lateral rectus muscle	Abducts
Facial nerve (CN VII)	Orbicularis muscle	Closes upper and lower lids
Sympathetic nerve	1. Müller's muscle	1. Elevates upper lid
	2. Pupil dilator muscle	2. Opens pupil in response to stress, "fight-or-flight," and adrenergic drugs
	3. Skin of lid	3. Sweat glands

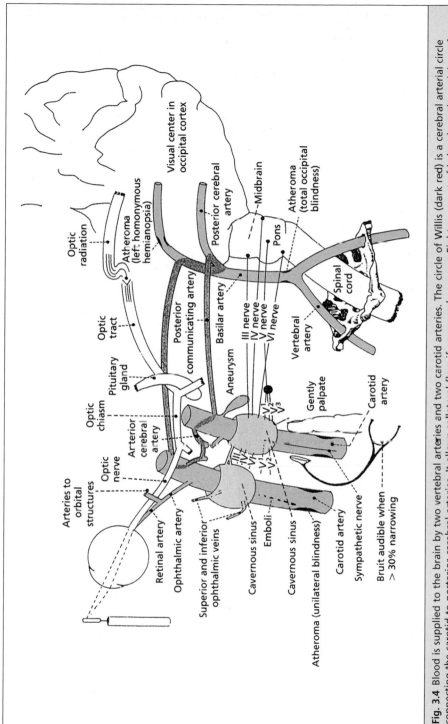

Fig. 3.4 Blood is supplied to the brain by two vertebral arteries and two carotid arteries. The circle of Willis (dark red) is a cerebral arterial circle connecting the carotid to posterior cerebral arteries. It allows collateral flow if one vessel narrows. Eighty percent of ischemic strokes originate from the carotid and 20% from the vertebral or basilar circulation.

Strabismus

Strabismus refers to the nonalignment of the eyes such that an object in space is not visualized simultaneously by the fovea of each eye.

If one eye is occluded while both eyes are fusing, the occluded eye may turn in (esophoria, noted with the letter E) or out (exophoria, X). Small phorias are usually asymptomatic. A phoria may degenerate into a tropia. A tropia is an eyeturn that occurs spontaneously. A tropia is more likely to occur as the amount of the phoria increases and as the patient's ability to compensate decreases. This occurs with tiredness later in the day and from any stimulus that dissociates the eyes, such as poor vision in one eye. Absence of a phoria (perfectly straight eyes) is termed orthophoria.

Complications of strabismus

1. Amblyopia

Also called lazy eye, amblyopia is decreased vision due to improper use of an eye in childhood. The two common causes are an eyeturn (strabismic amblyopia) or a refractive error (refractive amblyopia), uncorrected before age 8. In strabismus, children unconsciously suppress the deviated eye to avoid diplopia.

Types of tropias	
Esotropia (ET)	Deviation of eye nasally
Exotropia (XT)	Deviation of eye outward (temporally)
Hypertropia (HT)	Deviation of eye upward
Intermittent tropia	A phoria that spontaneously breaks to a tropia; indicate with parentheses. Example: R (ET) = right intermittent esotropia
Constant monocular tropia	Present at all times in one eye. Example: RXT, constant right exotropia. Often associated with loss of vision, if onset in childhood
Alternating tropia	Either eye can deviate. Vision is usually equal in both eyes

Strabismic amblyopia is treated by patching the good eye (Fig. 3.5), thereby forcing the child to use his amblyopic eye. The better eye is patched fulltime—one week for each year of age. It is repeated until there is no improvement on two consecutive visits. Refractive amblyopia is treated by correcting the refractive error with glasses and patching the better eye. Both types must be treated in early childhood because after age 5, it is difficult to improve vision. After age 8, improvement is almost impossible, but should be tried.

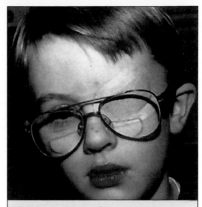

Fig. 3.5 Patching for amblyopia.

2. Poor cosmetic appearance

Tropias that cannot be corrected with spectacles may be cosmetically unacceptable and the patient may desire surgery.

3. Loss of fusion

Fusion occurs when the images from both eyes are perceived as one object, with resulting stereopsis (three-dimensional vision). Many patients with tropias never gain the ability to fuse. Finer grades of fusion are assessed by using the Wirt stereopsis test.

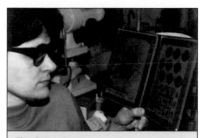

Fig. 3.6 Wirt stereopsis

Wirt stereopsis test (Fig. 3.6)

While wearing polarized glasses, the patient views a test card. The degree of fusion is determined by the number of pictures correctly described in three dimensions.

Near point of convergence (NPC) (Fig. 3.7)

The NPC is the closest point at which the eyes can cross to view a near object. It is measured by having the patient make a maximal effort to fixate on a small object as it is moved toward his or her eyes. The distance at which the eyes stop converging and one turns out is recorded as the NPC. Convergence insufficiency must be considered if the NPC is greater than 8 cm. These patients may complain of

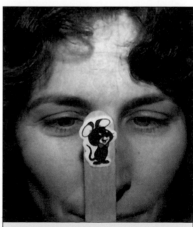

Fig. 3.7 Near point of convergence.

diplopia or other difficulties while reading. Exercises or prism glasses may help.

Accommodative esotropia
(Fig. 3.8)

When the lens of a normal eye focuses, it simultaneously causes the eyes to converge. Hyperopes not wearing glasses must focus the lens of their eye (accommodation) to see clearly near and far. This focusing stimulates the accommodative reflex causing convergence of the eyes. When the ratio of convergence to accommodation is abnormally high, an esotropia results, which corrects with lenses.

Nonaccommodative esotropia
(Figs 3.9–3.11)

This is due to a defect in the brain not related to the accommodative reflex. It is corrected by surgically weakening the medial rectus muscle by recessing its insertion posteriorly on the sclera or by tightening the lateral rectus muscle by resecting part of it. Less often, botulinum toxin is injected to weaken eye muscles.

An epicanthal skin fold connects the nasal upper and lower lids (Fig. 3.12) and is common in infants and Asians. It gives the false impression of a cross-eye called pseudostrabismus.

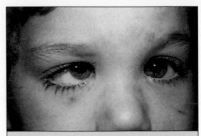

Fig. 3.8a Accommodative esotropia.

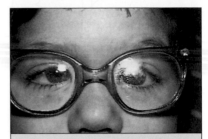

Fig. 3.8b Accommodative esotropia corrected with hyperopic lenses.

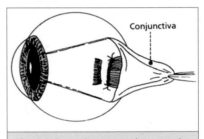

Fig. 3.9 Recession to weaken muscle.

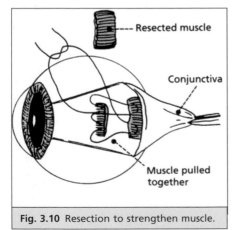

Fig. 3.10 Resection to strengthen muscle.

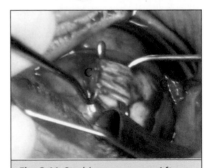

Fig. 3.11 Strabismus surgery: After incising the conjunctiva (C), the medial rectus m. is exposed and isolated with 2 muscle hooks. Courtesy of Elliot Davidoff, MD.

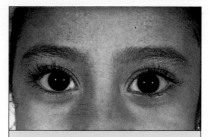

Fig. 3.12 Epicanthal folds causing false impression of cross-eye (pseudostrabismus)

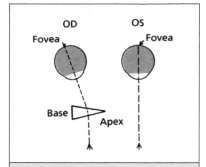

Fig. 3.13 Right esotropia neutralized with prism (apex-in).

Measurement of the amount of eye-turn with prisms

Ocular deviations are measured in prism diopters. When light passes through a prism, it is bent toward the base of the prism. One prism diopter (1 Δ) displaces the image 1 cm at a distance of 1 meter from the prism. Do not confuse prism diopters (Δ) with lens diopters (D).

In a right esotropia, the right fovea is turned temporally. To focus the light on the right fovea, a prism (apex in) is placed in front of the right eye (Fig. 3.13). For an exotropia, use apex out. *Rule:* point prism apex in the direction of the tropia.

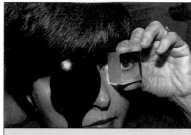

Fig. 3.14 Prism cover test.

Prism cover test for measurement of eye-turn (Fig. 3.14)

The patient fixates on an object at 20 ft. When the fixating eye is occluded, the deviated eye must move to look at the target. Increasing amounts of prism are placed in front of the deviated eye until no movement is noted when the cover is moved back and forth over each eye.

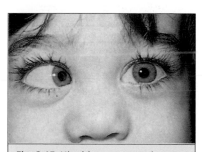

Fig. 3.15 Hirschberg: esotropia.

Hirschberg's test

When the cover test is difficult to perform on young children, the angle of strabismus can be estimated by using Hirschberg's test (Figs 3.15–3.17). As the child fixates on a point source of light, the position of the corneal light reflexes is noted. Each 1 mm of deviation

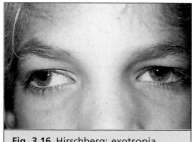

Fig. 3.16 Hirschberg: exotropia.

from the center of the cornea is equivalent to approximately 14 Δ of deviation. A reflex 2 mm temporal to the center of the cornea indicates an esotropia of approximately 28 Δ.

Causes of strabismus

1 Paralytic strabismus is due to cranial nerve (III, IV, or VI) disease or eye-muscle weakness from thyroid disease, traumatic contusions, myasthenia gravis, or orbital floor fractures.
2 Nonparalytic strabismus is due to a malfunction of a center in the brain. It is often inherited and begins in childhood.

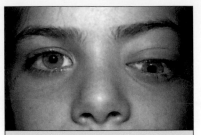

Fig. 3.17 Hirschberg: left hypotropia.

Demonstration of paralytic strabismus

In paralytic strabismus, the amount of deviation is greatest when gaze is directed in the field of action of the weakened muscle. To demonstrate underaction of any of the 12 external ocular muscles, the patient fixates on an object moved into each of the six cardinal fields of gaze (Fig. 3.18). Each position

Comparison of paralytic and nonparalytic strabismus

	Paralytic	Nonparalytic
Age of onset	Usually in older persons	Usually starts before 6 years of age
Complaint since	Diplopia	Cosmetic eye turn; less diplopia—child suppresses deviated eye
Eye turn	Largest deviation in field of action of affected muscle	No one muscle is underactive; deviation similar in all directions
Vision	Not affected	Deviated eye may have loss of vision (amblyopia)
Plan	Neurologic workup	Ophthalmic workup

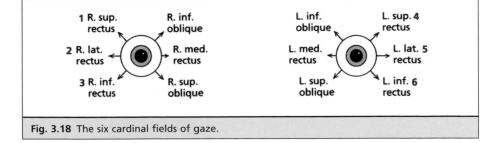

Fig. 3.18 The six cardinal fields of gaze.

tests one muscle of each eye (e.g., position 3 tests the right inferior rectus and the left superior oblique muscles). In addition to observing for underaction or overaction of the muscles, ask the patient where diplopia is greatest. For exact measurements, use the prism cover test.

Most often the cause for CN III, IV, and VI paralysis cannot be confirmed, since it is due to ischemia from small-vessel closure. Testing is done to rule out causes such as multiple sclerosis, aneurysms, neoplasms, and other rarer conditions, especially in younger individuals where vessel closure is not likely. Ischemia from diabetes is the most common cause and often resolves within 10 weeks.

Oculomotor nerve (CN III)

CN III paralysis (Figs 3.19–3.21) results in underaction of the inferior oblique and medial, inferior, and superior rectus muscles, resulting in an eye turned down and out. Since this nerve also innervates the levator palpebral muscle, which elevates the lid and the pupillary constrictor muscle, the lid is drooped and the pupil is dilated. CN III paralysis due to diabetes often spares the pupil.

Always examine for a dilated pupil after head trauma. CN III parallels the posterior communicating artery (see Figs 3.4 and 3.60) so that ruptured aneurysms in the circle of Willis are a common cause of paralysis with a dilated pupil and an explosive headache (Figs 3.22 and 3.23). Also, CN III passes under the tentorial ridge in the brain and is highly susceptible to uncal herniation of the brain. Herniation may follow increased intracranial pressure from cerebral edema, hematoma, tumor, abscess, or cerebral spinal fluid obstruction. Although a dilated pupil is a more common ominous sign after head injury, small or unequal pupils could indicate serious insults to other parts of the brain.

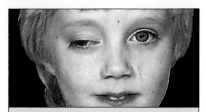

Fig. 3.19 Right CN III paralysis. In straight gaze, eye turns down and out with dilated pupil and ptosis.

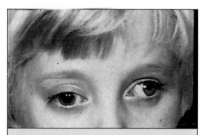

Fig. 3.20 Inability of right eye to look to the left due to medial rectus paralysis.

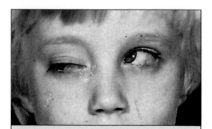

Fig. 3.21 Inability of right eye to look up to right due to superior rectus paralysis. Courtesy of David Taylor.

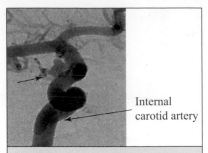

Internal
carotid artery

Fig 3.22 Cerebral angiogram of right carotid artery showing a 3 x 4 m posterior communicating a. aneurysm (↑). This occurred in a 50 year-old man with a subarachnoid hemorrhage and the worst headache of his life. Fifteen percent of patients with subarachnoid haemorrhages die before reaching the hospital.

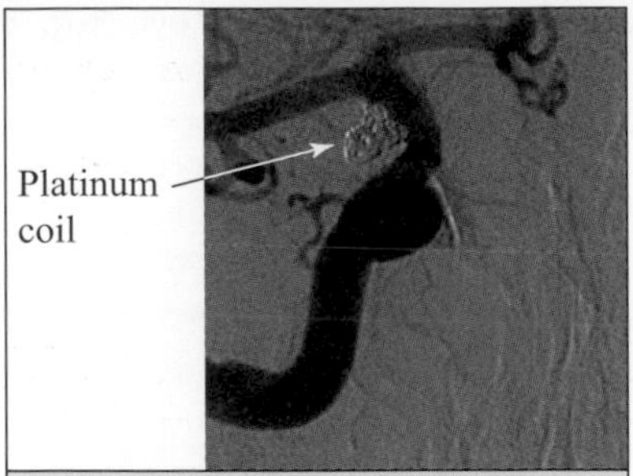

Platinum coil

Fig 3.23 Stent-assisted platinum coiling embolization of aneurysm. A small electric charge is sent to the linear platinum tip when it enters the aneurysm. This charge detaches it, causes folding, and promotes thrombosis. Courtesy of Stavropoula I Tjoumakaris, MD and Robert Rossenwasser, MD. Thomas Jefferson University Hospital Endovascular Neurological Surgery Dept.

Trochlear nerve (CN IV)

The trochlear nerve (CN IV) innervates the superior oblique muscle. Since this muscle acts as a depressor when the eye is rotated nasally, it causes patients to have vertical diplopia when looking down to read. Since intorsion is this muscle's main action, there is a head tilt to the opposite shoulder so that the eye doesn't have to be intorted (Fig. 3.24). If the doctor forces the patient's head straight (Fig. 3.25), the superior rectus must act as an intorter. Since the superior rectus also elevates the eye as it intorts, vertical diplopia occurs. A common cause of superior oblique muscle dysfunction is trauma since it passes through the trochlea (see Fig. 3.1), where it is accessible to injury due to its location just under the superior nasal orbital rim. All patients with a head tilt should be checked for trochlear nerve dysfunction.

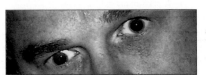

Fig. 3.24 Left superior oblique paralysis. To avoid diplopia, head is tilted to the opposite shoulder. Courtesy of Joseph Calhoun.

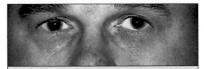

Fig. 3.25 Paralytic left superior oblique with vertical diplopia in primary gaze. Note: sclera visible below left cornea.

Abducens nerve (CN VI)

The abducens nerve (CN VI) innervates the lateral rectus muscle that abducts the eye. Loss of function causes diplopia and a cross-eye (Figs 3.26–3.28). As this nerve may be damaged from increased intracranial pressure, one should be alert to an associated headache, nausea, and papilledema.

Trigeminal nerve (CN V)

The trigeminal nerve (CN V) is the sensory nerve of the head and face (Fig. 3.29).

V_1: ophthalmic branch—sensory to upper lid, eye, and nose.

V_2: maxillary branch—sensory to lower lid and cheek.

V_3: mandibular branch—no ocular action.

Injury may cause an anesthetic effect, as occurs in an orbital blow-out fracture or pain as occurs in herpes zoster dermatitis (Fig. 3.30) or trigeminal neuralgia (tic douloureux).

Herpes zoster dermatitis (shingles) is due to reactivation of the latent varicella virus from an episode of chicken pox in childhood. It often affects the ophthalmic division of CN V. There may be an associated iritis, keratitis, a fever, and adenopathy. Rx: valacyclovir

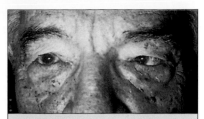

Fig. 3.26 Right lateral rectus paralysis in right gaze. Courtesy of Elliot Davidoff.

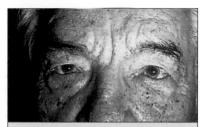

Fig. 3.27 Right lateral rectus paralysis, straight gaze.

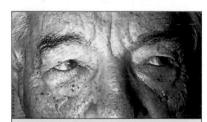

Fig. 3.28 Right lateral rectus paralysis, left gaze.

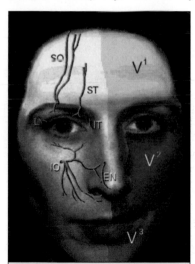

Fig. 3.29 The three divisions of the trigeminal nerve, V1, V2, V3 and the individual nerves SO, supraorbital; ST, supratrochlear; L, lacrimal; IT, infratrochlear; IO, infraorbital; EN, external nasal.

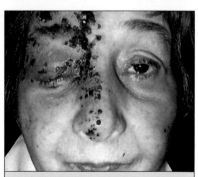

Fig. 3.30 Herpes zoster dermatitis. Think of shingles when the dermatitis follows the distribution of CN V and doesn't cross the facial midline.

(Valtrex) 1000 mg PO TID × 7 days. It must be started within 72 hrs of onset of skin lesions. The treatment for iritis is similar to the treatment for other causes of iritis. Post-herpetic neuralgia is the most common sequela. A 2010 study based on the entire population of Taiwan reports a ninefold increase in the risk of cancer the year following a diagnosis of herpes zoster ophthalmicus. The meaning of this relationship is not yet understood.

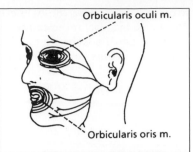

Fig. 3.31 Facial nerve to orbicularis oculi and oris muscles.

Facial nerve (CN VII)

The facial nerve (CN VII) innervates the orbicularis oculi muscle, which closes the lid, and also the muscles that control facial expression (Fig. 3.31). It also stimulates lacrimal secretion.

The common CN VII paralysis in adults is called Bell's palsy and is usually due to ischemia or a virus (Figs 3.32 and 3.33).

Minor eyelid spasms of the orbicularis muscle which the patient senses as a twitching of the muscles of the lid, and usually unnoticed by an observer, is called myokymia. It may be related to stress, fatigue, too much caffeine, or hyperthyroidism, and often disappears in weeks.

Blepharospasm (Fig. 3.34) is a more severe spasm of the orbicularis muscle causing the eyelids to close involuntarily. The first-line treatment is to give six injections of Botulinum toxin (Botox) into the muscles around the eye every 3–4 months. It blocks the release of acetylcholine at the neuro-muscular junction. Severe cases may require surgical removal of the muscle or seventh nerve.

Vestibulocochlear nerve (CN VIII)

The vestibulocochlear nerve (CN VIII) is the sensory nerve for hearing and balance. The vestibular branch has sensory fibers in the semi-circular canals and the vestibule of the inner ear. Their axons connect in a complex system to the nuclei of CN III, IV and VI in the brainstem. These nuclei control the muscles

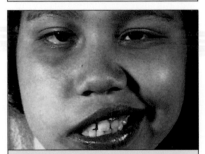

Fig. 3.32 Right CN VII paralysis causes decreased blinking and inability to close lids completely (see Fig. 6.12).

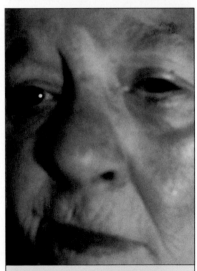

Fig. 3.33 In CN VII paralysis, the inability to close the eye causes corneal dessication. To remedy this, in the above patient, the left lateral upper and lower tarsus were sutured together (tarsorraphy). It may be temporary or permanent.

that move the eye. This vestibulo-ocular reflex maintains fixation and balance when the head moves. Diseases of this pathway cause nystagmus and the illusionary whirling sensation called vertigo. The cochlear division of this nerve is responsible for hearing.

Normal nystagmus

This is an involuntary rhythmic movement of the eyes in a horizontal, vertical, or rotary fashion. Pendular nystagmus means equal motion in each direction, while the jerky type has a quicker movement in one direction than the other. Fine movements are most easily seen by observing the retina with an ophthalmscope or at the slit lamp.

Vestibular nystagmus is due to stimulation of the semicircular canals of the ear, either by rotating the body or placing cold or hot water in the ear.

Optokinetic nystagmus is a jerky type of movement, as occurs when one watches scenery go by while riding in a car (Fig. 3.35). End-point nystagmus is a jerky type occurring in extreme positions of gaze.

Abnormal nystagmus

Diseases of the vestibular system, originating in the inner ear or in the cerebellum, are the most common reasons for vertigo with associated nystagmus. A clue in differentiating the cause of the vertigo and nystagmus is that CN VIII disease often has signs localizing it to the ear. Cerebellar disease often has impairment of speech and gait.

Gaze nystagmus occurs in certain fields of gaze. It is caused by drugs such as Dilantin or barbiturates, and in demyelinating diseases, cerebral vascular insufficiency, and brain tumors.
Infantile nystagmus syndrome has a pendular nystagmus starting at birth and usually causes reduced vision. If there is a position of gaze with less movement (null angle), eye muscle surgery or prisms may be tried to move this position to a straight-ahead gaze.

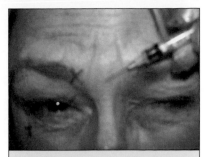

Fig. 3.34 Subcutaneous Botox is injected (X) into the underlying orbicularis oculi m. to treat blepharospasm. Care is taken not to inject the center of the upper lid so as to avoid the belly of the levator m. which would cause ptosis if paralyzed.

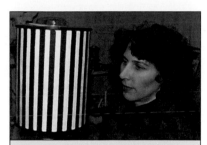

Fig. 3.35 Optokinetic drum that stimulates optokinetic nystagmus when rotated. Hysterics and malingerers faking total blindness cannot help but move their eyes.

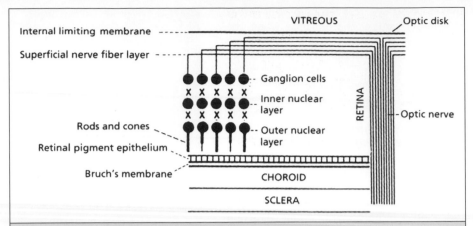

Internal limiting membrane

Superficial nerve fiber layer

VITREOUS

Optic disk

Ganglion cells

Inner nuclear layer

Outer nuclear layer

RETINA

Optic nerve

Rods and cones

Retinal pigment epithelium

Bruch's membrane

CHOROID

SCLERA

Fig. 3.36 Schematic cross section of retina. The ganglion cell fibers on the surface of the retina become covered with a myelin sheath at the optic disk and this continuation of these fibers outside the eye is then called the optic nerve.

Spasmus nutans is a unilateral or bilateral pendular nystagmus beginning at about 6 months of age and often ending by 2 years of age. It may be associated with head nodding.

Blindness from any cause that begins early in life may result in pendular nystagmus.

Optic nerve (CN II)

The optic nerve (CN II) is made up of 1.2 million retinal ganglion cell axons which transmit the visual message from the eye to the brain. The nerve begins at the optic disk (papilla) as the ganglion cell axons exit the eye (Figs 3.36 and 6.78).

When the intraocular ganglion cells or the extraocular optic nerve are damaged, the normal pink or orange optic disk may turn chalk white (Fig. 3.37).

In the case of glaucoma, the pallor is associated with excavation (cupping) of the disk (Fig. 3.38).

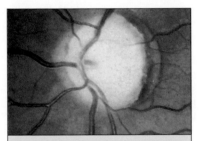

Fig. 3.37 Optic atrophy resulting from ischemia, transection, toxicity, or inflammation.

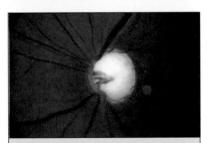

Fig. 3.38 Optic atrophy with cupping due to glaucoma.

Intraocular causes for loss of optic nerve fibers

Glaucoma is a disease of the optic nerve aggravated by high intraocular pressure. It is the most common cause of optic neuropathy. Therefore, a whole section is devoted to it (p. 87).

Retinal ischemia due to retinal artery and vein occlusion or diabetic closure of capillaries may cause loss of ganglion cells and result in pallor of the disk. Thinning of the ganglion cell layer also occurs in high myopia, retinitis pigmentosa, chorioretinitis, and numerous less common retinal diseases.

Extraocular causes for loss of optic nerve fibers

When the nerve near the optic disk is inflamed (optic neuritis), you may see papillitis with an ophthalmoscope. Signs of papillitis include flame hemorrhages around the disk, cells in the overlying vitreous, and a blurred disk margin (Fig. 3.39). Optic neuritis could cause dimming of vision, reduced central vision, decreased pupil reaction to light, reduced color vision, and pain with eye movement.

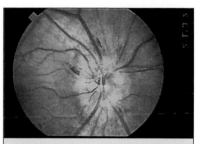

Fig. 3.39 Optic neuritis with papillitis.

When light is shined in a normal eye, both pupils constrict. This is called a consensual light reflex. Damage to the optic nerve (CN II) reduces direct pupillary constriction to light. The diseased eye will constrict well when light shines on the other eye due to the normal consensual reflex. Shining a light back and forth between eyes, called the swinging light test (Fig. 3.40), reveals the eye with optic atrophy to be dilating as the light shines on it since the stronger consensual reflex is wearing off. This is called a Marcus Gunn pupil and is helpful in diagnosing optic neuritis. Also in optic neuritis the patient claims the light is dimmer in the diseased eye as it is shined back and forth.

Fifty percent of cases of optic neuritis are due to multiple sclerosis. Multiple sclerosis is a

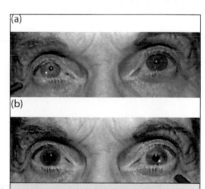

Fig. 3.40 Swinging light test. (a) Both pupils constrict when light shines in normal right eye due to consensual reflex. (b) Left pupil in eye with optic neuritis dilates as light shines on it, since consensual stimulation wears off.

chronic relapsing condition with a usual onset between the third and fifth decades. It has a partial autoimmune etiology that causes multiple areas of demyelination in the central nervous system (Fig. 3.41a). Diplopia due to CN III, IV or VI paralysis or decreased vision is often the first symptom of the disease. In multiple sclerosis, optic neuritis often occurs without papillitis due to the more posterior involvement of the nerve. Corticosteroids may shorten the length of time the optic neuritis lasts, but has little effect on the final loss of vision.

The next most common cause of optic neuritis is non-inflammatory (non-arteritic) ischemia due to arteriosclerosis. This commonly occurs in older patients and there is no firmly established treatment. In this elderly population, ischemia could have an inflammatory cause and one must always consider the possibility of giant cell arteritis (GCA) - also called temporal or cranial arteritis. Failure to recognize GCA early could result in bilateral blindness and even death. GCA almost always occurs after age 50 and the occurrence rises dramatically with each decade. Besides having symptoms typical of optic neuropathy patients may also have scalp tenderness, pain on chewing, arthritis, weight loss, loss of appetite and malaise. An elevated sedimentation rate and C-reactive protein with a positive temporal artery biopsy confirms the diagnosis. See Figs 3.41b-d:

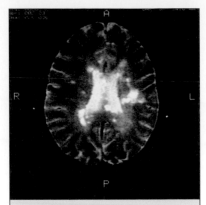

Fig. 3.41a Magnetic resonance imaging (MRI) of the brain. Areas of high intensity correspond to demyelinating plaques, which are present in 90% of known multiple sclerosis cases. MRI of orbit could show thickening of optic nerve when optic neuritis is present.

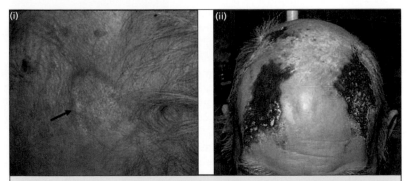

Fig. 3.41b Two of the clinical manifestations of cranial arteritis. (i) Photograph of an enlarged and nodular left temporal artery that is tender to palpation and pulseless. (ii) Haemorrhagic necrosis of the scalp in a patient with giant cell arteritis (GCA). Reprinted from Campbell et al. (2003). With permission from Blackwell Publishing Ltd.

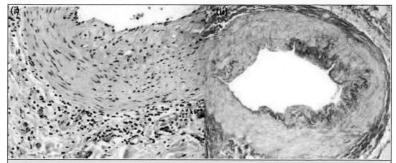

Fig. 3.41c Histopathologic examination of a temporal artery biopsy in a patient with giant cell arteritis (GCA). (i) Haematoxylin and eosin stain shows lymphocytic infiltration of the adventitia. (ii) Elastic tissue stain shows fragmentation of the internal elastic lamina and intimal hyperplasia.

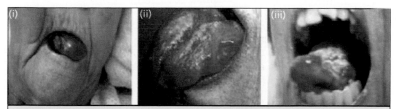

Fig. 3.41d Three examples of ischaemic oral lesions caused by giant cell arteritis (GCA). (i) Patient with tongue and lip infarction. (ii) Cyanosis and oedema in the tongue. (iii) A necrotic lesion of the tongue. From Goicochea M, Correale J, Bonamico L et al. (2007): Tongue necrosis in temporal arteritis. *Headache* **47**: 1213–1215, with permission from Blackwell Publishing Ltd.

Prompt treatment with high doses of steroids should be administered even if the biopsy cannot be performed for several days.

The pupil

Both pupils are equally round and approximately 3–4 mm in diameter. Anisocoria refers to a difference in pupil size, and 4% of normal people may have as much as 1 mm of difference. Miosis is a constricted pupil, and mydriasis is a dilated pupil. Pupil size is determined by a dilator muscle controlled by the sympathetic nerve and a constrictor muscle that has cholinergic innervation via CN III (Fig. 3.42).

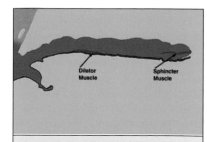

Fig. 3.42 Radial fibers of dilator muscle and ring of constrictor muscle near pupillary margin. Courtesy of Pfizer Pharmaceuticals.

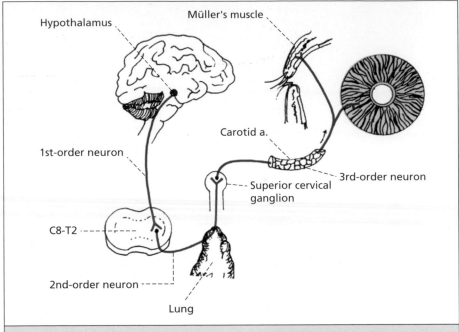

Fig. 3.43 Sympathetic pathway.

Hypothalamus

Müller's muscle

1st-order neuron

Carotid a.

3rd-order neuron

Superior cervical ganglion

C8-T2

2nd-order neuron

Lung

Less common causes of optic neuropathy include drug or tobacco or alcohol toxicity, folic acid or vitamin B12 deficiency, tumors, or thyroid disease. Infections such as mumps, measles, and influenza rarely may be associated.

Sympathetic nerve

The iris dilator muscle and the Müller's muscle that elevates the lid are both stimulated by the sympathetic nerve that begins in the hypothalamus (Fig. 3.43) and descends down the spinal column. At C8–T2 it synapses and then exits and passes over the apex of the lung. It ascends in the neck until it synapses, and follows the carotid artery into the skull and orbit. It dilates the pupil in response to the "fight or flight" stimulus. Damage to this nerve causes Horner's syndrome (Fig. 3.44): miosis, ptosis, and decreased sweating (anhidrosis).

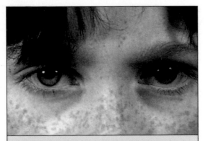

Fig. 3.44 Right Horner's syndrome. Associated pain on the same side is highly suggestive of a dissection of the wall of the carotid artery and should be referred immediately to the emergency room for vascular imaging. If caught early, anticoagulation may prevent a stroke. (see Figs 3.45 and 3.46)

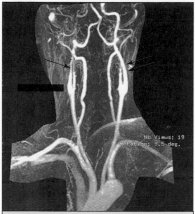

Fig 3.45 Carotid artery dissection: Magnetic resonance angiography (MRA) of right internal carotid (↑) shows decreased blood flow. Left internal carotid artery is normal (↑↑).

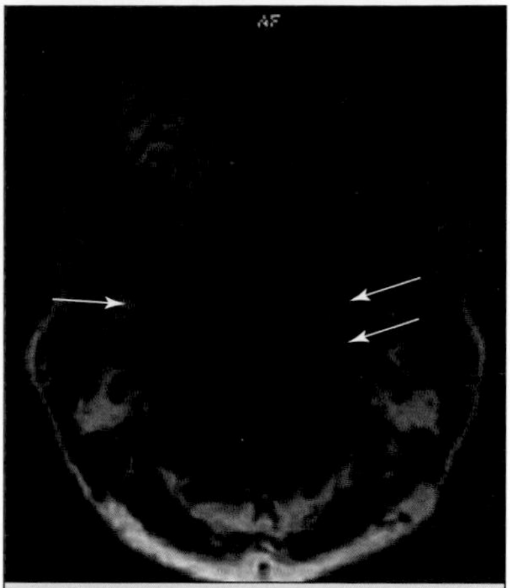

Fig. 3.46 MRA shows right wall hematoma seen on the black blood image (↑) and is compatible with a right carotid dissection. Left carotid is normal (↑↑).

Pupillary light reflex (Fig. 3.47)

Light shining on the retina stimulates the optic nerve and then the optic chiasm and optic tract. Here, it exits from the visual pathway to stimulate the Edinger–Westphal nucleus in the midbrain. The pupillary fibers leave the nucleus and travel with CN III until it synapses at the ciliary ganglion in the orbit. It innervates the iris sphincter muscle. Light shining in one eye causes that pupil and the pupil of the other eye to simultaneously constrict. The latter is referred to as the consensual light reflex. Both pupils also constrict when the eye accommodates from distance to near. This normal state may be noted as PERRLA—pupils equally round and reactive to light and accommodation. An MRI of the brain, neck, and upper chest should be considered when Horner's syndrome occurs in children to rule out neuroblastomas when there are no other obvious causes such as birth trauma.

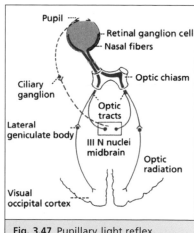

Fig. 3.47 Pupillary light reflex.

Causes of Horner's syndrome	
Neuron I	Spinal cord trauma, tumors, demyelinating disease, syringomyelia
Neuron II	Apical lung tumors, goiter, neck injury, or surgery
Neuron III	Carotid dissections, migraine, cavernous sinus, or orbital disease

Causes of irregular pupils

Size of pupil

○ 3 ○ 4 ○ 5 ○ 6 ○ 7 ○ 8 ○ 9 ○ 10

	Miosis		Mydriasis	
↑ *Cholinergic*	↓ *Sympathetic*	*Irritation to constrictor muscle*	↓ *Cholinergic*	↑ *Sympathetic*
Pilocarpine drops used for glaucoma	Horner's syndrome	Iritis	Atropine	Phenylephrine
Morphine	Aldomet	Histamine release from inflammation	CN III paralysis	Epinephrine
	Reserpine		Adie's pupil	Anxiety
			Antihistamines	Cocaine
				Decongestants

Damaged constrictor muscle
High eye pressure >40 mmHg
Trauma (especially common with hyphemas)

Adie's pupil (tonic pupil)

This is a dilated pupil with a reduced direct and consensual light reflex. It reacts slowly to accommodation, and eventually becomes smaller and stays smaller than the other eye, hence the name tonic pupil. It is due to a benign defect in the ciliary ganglion (Fig. 3.47). Resulting denervation hypersensitivity causes the tonic pupil to constrict intensely compared with the other eye in response to one drop of weak pilocarpine 1/10%.

Visual field testing

The field of vision of each eye extends to 170° in the horizontal and 130° in the vertical meridian. Routine testing of vision with a Snellen chart recorded as 20/20 only means that the central few degrees corresponding to the macula are normal.

1 Amsler grid. This hand-held black cross-hatched card tests the central 20° of the visual field. Waviness of lines is called metamorphopsia, and is characteristic of a wrinkled retina from macular disease (Fig. 3.48 and Appendix 2).

2 A tangent screen is a sheet of black felt (Fig. 3.49). It measures the central 60° of field. The patient is seated 1 or 2 meters from the screen, with one eye occluded. The examiner moves a small white ball centrally until the patient first sees it. Areas blind to this small object are tested with progressively larger objects.

3 Hemisphere perimeters (Fig. 3.50) test the entire 170° of horizontal field and 130° of vertical field. Automated perimeters are expensive but save examiners' time and gives record of field. Static perimeters project increasingly intense stimuli at one location until it is first seen.

4 Confrontation testing is used when instruments aren't available. The patient is seated opposite the examiner. The patient closes his or her right eye; the examiner closes his or her own left eye, and each fixates on the other's open eye. The examiner moves an

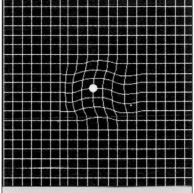

Fig. 3.48 Amsler grid. Distortion in macular degeneration.

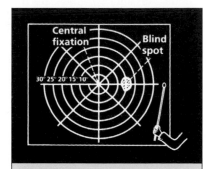

Fig. 3.49 Tangent screen central 60°. It is useful when patients cannot perform the more difficult automated perimetry.

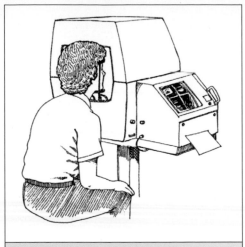

Fig. 3.50 Automated hemisphere perimeter tests central and peripheral fields.

object in from the periphery and it should be seen simultaneously by both individuals. This technique compares patient's and examiner's field.

Scotomas due to ocular and optic nerve disease

A scotoma is loss of part of the field. Relative scotomas are areas of visual field blind to small objects, but able to perceive larger stimuli. Absolute scotomas are totally blind areas.

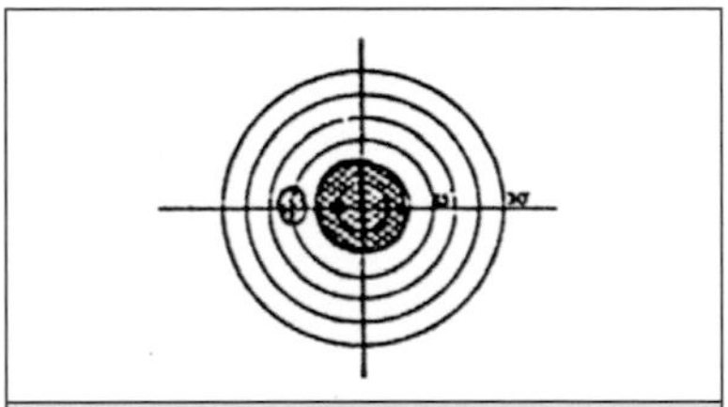

The normal blind spot is an absolute scotoma located 15° temporal to central fixation, which corresponds to the normal absence of rods and cones on the optic disk. It is plotted first (Fig. 3.51). If the blind spot cannot be located, the test is considered unreliable.

Central scotomas (Fig. 3.52) occur in macular degeneration. Central and paracentral scotomas (Fig. 3.53) are most characteristic of optic nerve disorders.

Unilateral altitudinal scotomas are defects above or below the horizontal meridian and are caused by an occlusion of a superior or

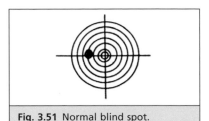

Fig. 3.51 Normal blind spot.

Fig. 3.52 Central scotoma.

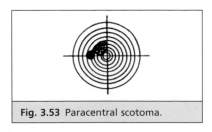

Fig. 3.53 Paracentral scotoma.

inferior retinal artery or vein and retinal detachments (Fig. 3.54).

Scotomas due to brain lesions

Field defects help to localize the site of brain lesions. Light focused on the temporal retina passes through the optic nerve and stimulates the occipital cortex on the same side, whereas fibers carrying impulses from the nasal retina cross over in the optic chiasm and stimulate the brain on the opposite side (Fig. 3.55). Therefore, defects at or posterior to the chiasm cause loss of vision in both eyes and respect the vertical meridian. If the defects are equal and on the same side, they are called homonymous (1, 4, 5). If they are unequal on the same side, they are termed incongruous (3). If they are on opposite sides in each eye, they are referred to as bitemporal or binasal (2).

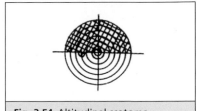

Fig. 3.54 Altitudinal scotoma.

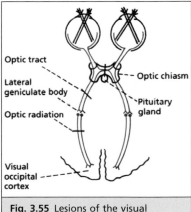

Optic tract
Lateral geniculate body
Optic radiation
Optic chiasm
Pituitary gland
Visual occipital cortex

Fig. 3.55 Lesions of the visual pathway.

1		The right homonymous hemianopsia is due to a lesion of the left occipital cortex.
2		In the optic chiasm the nasal axons from each eye cross over (Fig. 3.55). Pituitary tumors (Fig. 3.56) press on these fibers and cause a bitemporal hemianopsia. Since the pituitary is also below the optic chiasm, the inferior-nasal fibers are more often affected. Bilateral superior-temporal defects are, therefore, most common.
3		Optic tract lesions cause incongruous hemianopsia, that is, unequal in each eye.
4		Optic radiation defects are often partial because the fibers are so widespread. A parietal lobe tumor that damages the superior half of the left radiation, causes a right homonymous inferior quadrantopsia.
5		Occipital cortex lesions usually cause a partial homonymous hemianopsia that is often vascular in origin, but tumors, trauma, and abscesses are also common (Figs 3.4 and 3.57)

Color vision

Color vision depends on the ability to see three primary colors: red, green, and blue. Partial defects are inherited in 7% of males and 0.5% of females and are detected using Ishihara or American optical pseudoisochromatic plates. Loss of color vision could limit one's ability to become an electrician, airline pilot, or other profession requiring color discrimination. Acquired color defects may be due to retinal or visual pathway disease, the most common of which is optic neuritis. In acquired cases, test each eye separately and look for differences.

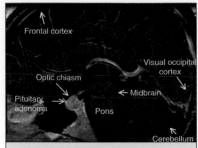

Fig. 3.56 CT scan of pituitary adenoma pressing on the optic chiasm which lies anterior and superior to it. Courtesy of Sandip Basak, MD.

Circulatory disturbances affecting vision (Refer to Fig. 3.4)

The blood supply to the brain originates from the two carotid arteries in the anterolateral neck and the two vertebral arteries passing through the cervical vertebrae. Transient loss of vision in those persons younger than age 50 is often due to a migrainous spasm of a cerebral artery. This causes scintillating scotomas (Fig. 3.57), which are brief flashes of light and/or zigzag lines that may precede a headache. It may progress to a homonymous hemianopsia lasting for 15–20 minutes.

If neurologic symptoms persist, they should go to the emergency room.

In older persons, the transient blurring is more often due to arteriosclerosis and is referred to as a transient ischemic attack (TIA). These visual obscurations—also called

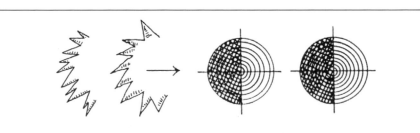

Fig. 3.57 Scintillating scotoma from migraine progressing to a left homonymous hemianopsia.

ministrokes—are caused by cholesterol, fibrin, or calcific emboli liberated from plaques, most often in the carotid artery. Symptoms occur as these emboli pass through the eye or visual cortex of the brain and usually last less than a half hour but could last up to 24 hours. If it lasts longer, it could turn into a permanent obstruction called a stroke.

Five percent of TIAs go on to develop a stroke within a month. So even if the symptoms have already cleared by the time the patient reaches your office, they should be cautioned about the risks of a permanent stroke and advised to see their primary care physician within a short time. If the TIA is still occurring after your examination, they should be sent directly to the emergency room since it could progress to a stroke. Eighty percent of strokes are ischemic and twenty percent are hemorrhagic. In the ER, they can be thoroughly evaluated to see if they meet the stringent guidelines to receive tissue plasminogen activator (tPA). There is a three hour therapeutic window from the onset of ischemic symptoms to administer this thrombolytic drug which could increase the chance of recovery from a stroke by 30–50% (Fig. 3.58). A CT scan is usually performed first in the emergency room to be sure it is ischemic and not hemorrhagic. Only then can tPA be safely administered.

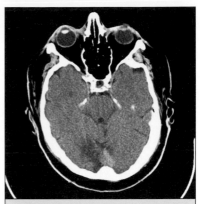

Fig. 3.58 MRI of right occipital infarct. Courtesy of Rand Kirtland, MD.

Tests for decreased circulation

A non-invasive duplex ultrasonography could show carotid stenosis and decreased blood flow. If positive, a CT angiogram may be ordered. Invasive arterial catheter angiography is infrequently used since there is a 1% chance of procedure-related stroke (Fig. 3.59), but it is still the gold standard. Carotid endarterectomy is performed in symptomatic (high risk) patients with 50% narrowing or in asymptomatic patients with 70% stenosis (see Appendix 2).

The right and left cavernous sinuses in the brain drain the superior and inferior

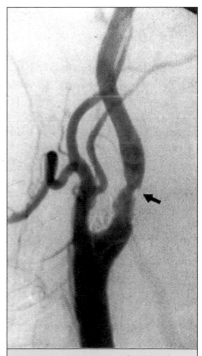

Fig. 3.59 Arteriogram of internal carotid artery narrowing.

	Carotid circulation	*Posterior cerebral circulation*
Cause	Cardiac abnormalities or carotid atheromas cause emboli to the retina and brain	Neck disorders affecting vertebral artery or emboli from atheroma
Symptoms	Unilateral curtain lasting a few minutes (amaurosis fugax): rarely headache, confusion, contralateral hemiparesis	Hemianopsia in both eyes: usually history of headache, dizziness, diplopia, drop attacks, or ringing in ears
Tests	An audible bruit over carotid artery in neck, duplex ultrasound, CT arteriogram, and cardiac evaluation	CT scan and MRI of brain (Fig. 3.58) with cardiac evaluation
Rx	Immediate thrombolysis (tPA), anticoagulants, endarterectomy or stenting less often	Immediate thrombolysis (tPA), anticoagulants or stent

ophthalmic veins from the orbit and face. Passing through the sinuses are the internal carotid artery, cranial nerves III–VI, and the sympathetic nerve (Fig. 3.60).

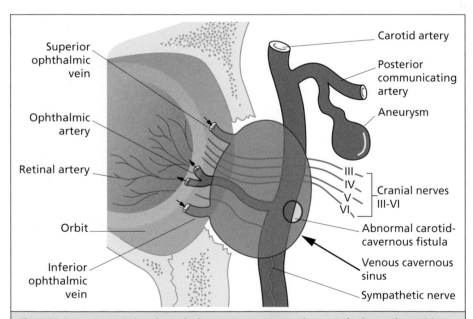

Fig. 3.60 Structures passing through the venous cavernous sinus are the internal carotid artery, cranial nerves (CN) III–VI, sympathetic nerve, superior and inferior ophthalmic veins, retinal and ophthalmic arteries. Note the two abnormalities. 1. carotid-cavernous fistula and 2. the posterior communicating artery with its aneurysm pressing on the cranial nerve III.

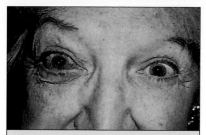

Fig. 3.61 Carotid cavernous fistula.

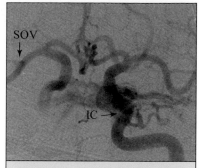

Fig. 3.62 Carotid cavernous fistula causing bilateral VI CN palsies. Contrast injection into the femoral artery showing an enlarged superior ophthalmic vein (SOV) with retrograde flow and internal carotid a. (IC) within cavernous sinus).

Carotid-cavernous fistulas usually result from trauma to an aneurysm of the carotid artery in the cavernous sinus (Figs 3.60 and 3.61). It connects high-pressure arterial to low-pressure venous circulation causing a pulsating exophthalmos with a bruit over the eye, and tortuous —"corkscrew" — conjunctival vessels. Diagnosis is confirmed with carotid arteriography that shows an enlarged superior ophthalmic vein draining in a retrograde way towards the orbit, instead of towards the cavernous sinus.

It must be distinguished from a cavernous sinus thrombosis which causes a non-pulsatile exophthalmos. The latter is often due to infection carried to the sinus via the superior and inferior ophthalmic veins. An MRI is useful to show widening of the cavernous sinus. A carotid-cavernous fistula and a cavernous sinus thrombosis are two causes of exophthalmos that can mimic orbital cellulitis (see Fig. 3.62). What both conditions have in common with orbital cellulitis are conjunctival vascular engorgement and chemosis (see Fig. 3.63); lids that are often swollen shut; and possible involvement of cranial nerves III–VI and the sympathetic nerve. Orbital cellulitis is usually unilateral; cavernous sinus thrombosis is commonly bilateral; and carotid-cavernous fistula is unilateral unless there are large connections between the right and left sinuses.

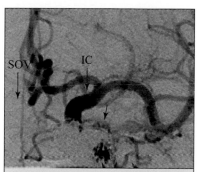

Fig. 3.63 Cerebral angiography through a femoral artery injection and passage of detachable platinum embolization coil through the superior ophthalmic vein located by a cutdown incision near the skinfold of the upper lid. Note the successful clouding of the obliterated cavernous sinus [up arrow] due to thrombosis and a narrowed SOV and uninterrupted blood flow through the distal internal carotid artery (IC) as it exits the sinus. Courtesy of Stavropoula I. Tjumakaris, MD and Robert Rosenwaisen, MD. Thomas Jefferson University Hospital, Cerebrovascular Neurological Surgery Dept.

Chapter 4
External structures

Begin with the four Ls: lymph, lacrimal, lashes, and lids.

Lymph nodes

Lymphatics from the lateral conjunctiva drain to the preauricular nodes just anterior to the ear. The nasal conjunctiva drains to the submandibular nodes (Fig. 4.1). Enlarged or tender nodes help to distinguish infectious from allergic lid and conjunctival inflammations.

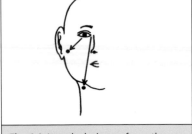

Fig. 4.1 Lymph drainage from the eye.

Lacrimal system

The tear film is made up of an outer oily component, a middle watery layer, and a deep mucous layer (Fig. 4.2).

An abnormality of any of these three components could cause symptoms such as dryness, grittiness, or sore eyes. The integrity

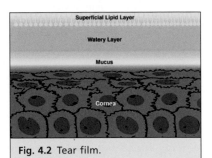

Fig. 4.2 Tear film.

Tear film

Type	Source (Fig. 4.5)	Common causes for decrease
Oily	Meibomian glands at edge of eyelid (Fig. 4.3)	Meibomian gland dysfunction is reported to be present in up to 86% of patients with documented dry eye.
Watery	Constant secretion by conjunctival glands and reflex secretion by the lacrimal gland in response to ocular irritation or emotion. In this reflex, CN V is the afferent pathway and CN VII is the efferent pathway	Normal decrease with age, especially in women after menopause. It is common in autoimmune diseases such as rheumatoid arthritis and lupus; after LASIK surgery; and from numerous drugs.
Mucous	Conjunctival goblet cells	Damaged conjunctiva in Stevens-Johnson syndrome (Fig. 1.9); ocular pemphigoid, and vitamin A deficiency (Fig. 4.8).

Manual for Eye Examination and Diagnosis, Eighth edition. Mark Leitman.
© 2012 John Wiley & Sons, Ltd. Published 2012 by John Wiley & Sons, Ltd.

of the tear film layer is estimated by the tear break up test TBUT (Fig. 4.4).

With most external eye infections, the tear film is highly infectious. In AIDS, only bloody tears are so far considered infectious. In any case, wash your hands between patient examinations.

With each blink (once every 4 seconds) acting as a lacrimal pump, the tear is moved nasally, where it enters the puncta and flows through the canaliculus, lacrimal sac, and the naso-lacrimal duct (NLD) into the nose (Fig. 4.5). All eye drops are more effective and have less systemic side effects if patients press on the puncta and close the eyes for 60 seconds. This minimizes flow into the nose. (Fig. 4.7)

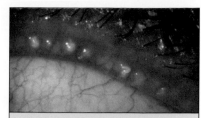

Fig. 4.3 There are 22 meibomian glands in both the upper and lower lid that normally secrete a clear, oily, meibum. In this case, the glands are dysfunctional with a white, pasty, discharge. Courtesy of Michael Lemp, MD.

Dry eye

Tear production normally decreases with age and could result in a symptomatic dry eye (keratoconjunctivitis sicca). It affects 20 million Americans.

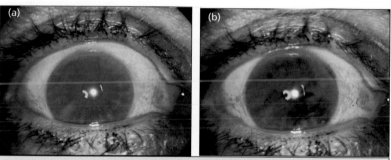

Fig. 4.4 Tear break up time (TBUT). (a) Fluorescein placed on a normal cornea and observed with cobalt blue light has a uniform appearance. (b) With the lids held open, the pattern may abnormally break up before 10 seconds. Courtesy of Elliot Davidoff, MD

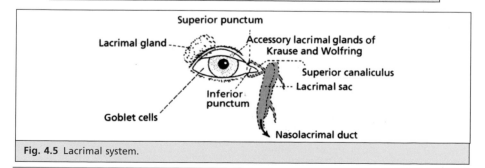

Fig. 4.5 Lacrimal system.

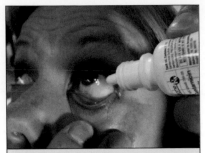

Fig. 4.6 Patients instill drop by holding bottle like a pencil with one hand while the other hand pulls lower lid down as they look up. It is even easier if patient lies down to stabilize the head, but some prefer to look in a mirror.

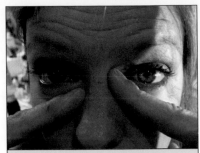

Fig. 4.7 After instilling drop, have patient push on upper and lower punctum for 60 seconds. This minimizes systemic side effects from drug entering nose and maximizes eye contact. Ask patient to show you their technique. The picture above demonstrates the correct technique on the left side.

Dryness may also occur from medications such as anticholinergics, tranquilizers, antihistamines, diuretics, or vitamin A deficiency. The latter may occur due to poor diet or malabsorption, which is increasing in incidence with the surging popularity of gastric bypass surgery used to treat obesity (Fig. 4.8). Loss of vision from vitamin A deficiency may result from dessication of the cornea due to dryness or from decreased function of the rod receptors in the retina, which requires this vitamin to produce the visual pigment rhodopsin. Paradoxically, excess Vitamin A is also toxic and can cause elevated intracranial pressure (pseudotumor cerebri) with significant loss of vision (Fig. 7.18 and p.127).

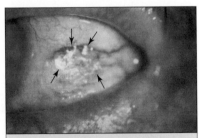

Fig. 4.8 White Bitot's spots (↑) on the conjunctiva due to vit. A deficiency following hemicolectomy. These white, keratinized lesions appear in the perilimbal area. Reprinted by permission from Macmillan Publishers *Eye*, Vol. 17, No. 5, 2003.

Dry eye also occurs in autoimmune diseases such as rheumatoid arthritis, lupus, and Sjögren's syndrome (dry eye, arthritis, dry mouth). In these cases, the lacrimal gland is immunologically damaged. Patients with Sjögren's have an increased chance of developing lymphoma. Blepharitis may cause dry eye due to meibomian gland dysfunction.

The Schirmer test measures tears on the surface of the eye. A drop of anesthetic is instilled and a strip of folded filter paper is placed inside the lateral lid (Fig. 4.9). Less than 10 mm of moist paper in 5 minutes is

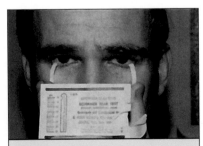

Fig. 4.9 Schirmer test.

presumptive of a dry eye. Patients with dry eye have an abnormal Schirmer test 21% of the time; central corneal staining with fluorescein 50% of the time (Fig. 6.11); and an abnormal tear break up time in 60% of cases (Fig. 4.4).

Dry eye is treated in the daytime with artificial tears and at night with ointments. There are many on the market. They vary mostly by their viscosity and whether they have preservatives. The patient often decides which one is best. Unfortunately, symptomatic relief lasts only 10–15 minutes, often leading to excessive use. In severely dry eyes, the puncta may be closed with punctal plugs (Fig. 4.10) or cautery to conserve tears. Room humidifiers may be tried and oral flaxseed oil increases meibomian gland secretions. Restasis (cyclosporine ophthalmic emulsion) 0.05% eye drops used twice a day may increase tear production in patients with keratoconjunctivitis sicca (chronic dry eye) whose tear production is suppressed due to inflammation of the goblet cells or lacrimal gland.

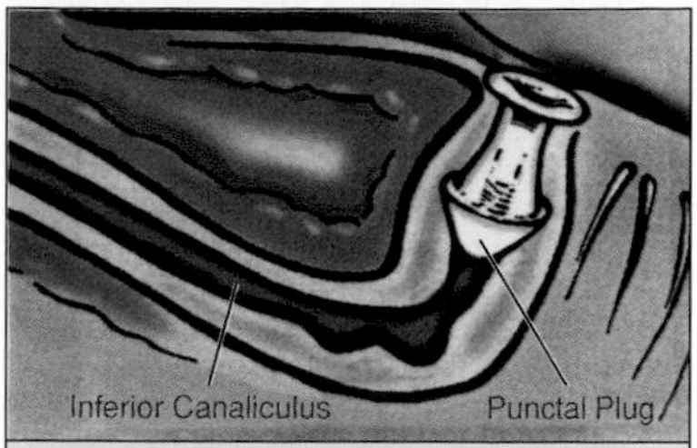

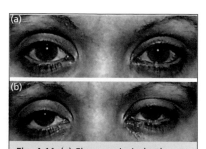

Inferior Canaliculus   Punctal Plug

Fig. 4.10 Punctal plug. A side effect of these plugs is stagnation of the tear film that can aggravate blepharitis by keeping the toxins and bacteria in prolonged contact with the surface of the eyes. Courtesy of EagleVision.

Tearing (epiphora)

Tearing is a very common complaint and often is minor enough so as not to require the work-up and treatment discussed below.

There are two causes of epiphora (tearing):
1 increased tear production due to emotion or eye irritation; or
2 normal tear production that cannot flow properly into the nose.

Tearing due to failure of drainage system

Once emotion and irritation are ruled out as the cause of tearing, an evaluation is made of the patency of the ducts leading into the nose. An obstruction is presumed if fluorescein dye placed on the conjunctiva (Fig. 4.11) disappears slowly and asymmetrically from one eye, or runs over the lid onto the cheek.

(a)

(b)

Fig. 4.11 (a) Fluorescein in both eyes. (b) Obstruction prevents exit of dye in left eye.

A - Failure of the tear to reach the puncta

This could be due to horizontal laxity of the lower lid which decreases the pumping action of the blink reflex, or an everted puncta, as occurs in an ectropion (Fig. 4.23), in which case, the tear lake is not in contact with the punctal orifice. Either can often be corrected by surgically tightening the lower lid with a full-thickness wedge resection.

B - Obstruction at the puncta or canaliculus

The puncta and canaliculi may become narrowed due to aging, topical drugs, trauma, and infections, especially from blepharitis.

The canaliculi can be dilated with progressively wider diameter punctal probes (Fig. 4.12b). If the lumen is still inadequate, a self-retaining bicanalicular stent (Fig. 4.13) can be inserted in the office with topical anesthetic and be left in place for three months. Traumatic laceration of the canaliculus can be repaired using a pigtail probe (Figs 4.12c and 4.14a). The probe is passed through the upper puncta toward the laceration. A silicone tube is threaded onto it and it is withdrawn. The probe is then passed through the lower puncta and the other end of the silicone tube is threaded onto it and it is withdrawn forming a continuous lumen to heal over the tube.

Rarely, the canaliculus can be obstructed from *Actinomyces israelii* infection. In this case, incise canaliculus; remove sand-like concretions. It is sensitive to penicillin and sulfa drugs.

C - Tearing due to nasolacrimal duct obstructions

In adults, it is often due to chronic nasal inflammation or aging. In infants, the distal opening of this duct in the nose—called the valve of Hasner—fails to open at birth. Although 90% spontaneously open by one year of age, repeated infections may mandate treatment at 6-12 months. In these infants, the puncta may be irritated and or probed to

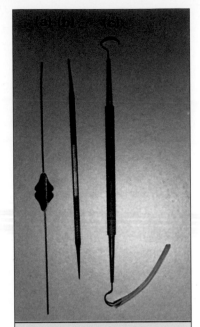

Fig. 4.12 (a) Punctal probe. (b) Punctum dilator. (c) Pigtail probe.

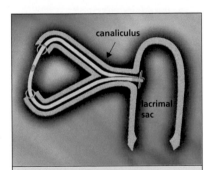

canaliculus

lacrimal sac

Fig. 4.13 Bicanalicular stent–for puncta stenosis or canalicular-constriction. Courtesy of FCI Ophthalmics.

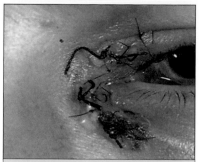

Fig. 4.14a Repair of canalicular tear.

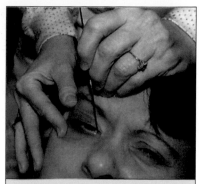

Fig. 4.15 Probing of nasolacrimal duct.

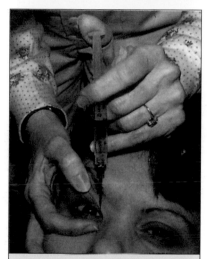

Fig. 4.14b Irrigation of nasolacrimal duct.

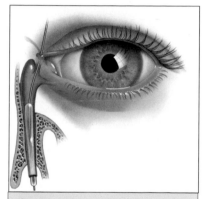

Fig. 4.16 Balloon catheter dacroplasty: inflate the balloon with sterile saline. Courtesy Quest Medical, Inc.

the nose (Figs 4.14b and 15). The same technique can be used in adults. If it is still narrowed, a balloon catheter may be used to widen the passage (Fig. 4.16), and/or a silicone stent may be inserted through the puncta, canaliculus, and nasolacrimal duct into the nose and left in place for 2–4 months.

If it still remains closed, a new surgical opening in the nasal bone is created and the mucosa of the lacrimal sac is sutured to the nasal mucosa (dacryocystorhinostomy). Besides tearing, an additional motivation for performing the latter surgical procedure is recurring infections of the lacrimal sac (dacryocystitis; Fig. 4.17) caused by stagnant tear flow.

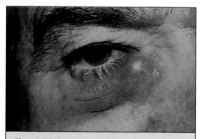

Fig. 4.17 Dacryocystitis.

Signs of dacryocystitis are swelling and tenderness over the lacrimal sac with pus exuding from the puncta when pressure is applied to the sac. Rx: massage the sac; nasal decongestant; local and systemic antibiotics; then a dacryocystorhinostomy to open the NLD.

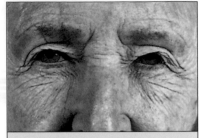
Fig. 4.18 Shriveled skin following allergy.

Lids

Lid swelling is commonly due to allergy, in which case the edema clears with a telltale shriveling of the skin between episodes (Fig. 4.18). Dependent edema caused by body fluid retention affects the lids on awakening and the ankles later in the day. Hypothyroidism (myxedema) and orbital venous congestion due to orbital masses or cavernous sinus thrombosis or fistulas are less common causes of edematous lids.

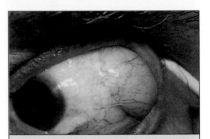
Fig. 4.19 Dermatochalasis.

Dermatochalasis is loose skin (Fig. 4.19) due to aging, and is aggravated by recurrent bouts of lid edema. There may be palpable orbital fat that herniated through the orbital septum (see Figs 4.21 and 4.27). A surgical blepharoplasty is performed for cosmetic reasons or if resulting drooping of the lid (ptosis) obstructs vision.

Lid-margin lacerations must be carefully approximated to prevent notching. Pass a 4-0 silk suture through both edges of the tough tarsal plate using the gray line for accurate alignment (Fig. 4.22).

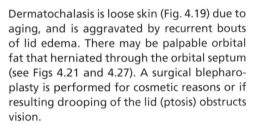
Fig. 4.20 Orbital fat under conjunctiva.

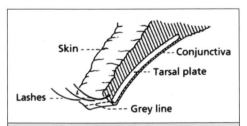
Fig. 4.22 Lid margin. The gray line delineates the mucocutaneous junction.

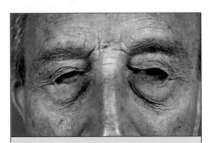
Fig. 4.21 Prolapsed fat through septum is palpable under skin.

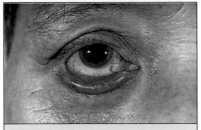

Fig. 4.23 Ectropion.

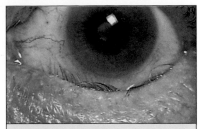

Fig. 4.24 Entropion.

An ectropion (Fig. 4.23a.) is an outturned lid. It is often caused by senile relaxing of the lid. This is aggravated in patients who chronically dab their tears or apply eye drops since both cause downward tugging and weakening of lid tissue. Less common causes are CN VII paralysis or traction of scarred skin on the lower lid. Correct with surgery.

An entropion (Fig. 4.24) is an inturned lid margin. It may be due to contraction of scarred conjunctiva (Figs 1.9 and 6.53a) senile lid laxity, or spasm of the orbicularis oculi muscle. It is corrected with surgery.

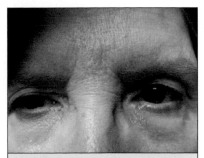

Fig. 4.25 Lid retraction in Grave's disease, causing the left eye to appear larger.

The palpebral fissure is the space between the upper and lower lid (Fig. 4.25). Differences in the size of the palpebral fissures occur with ptosis (droopy lid), lid retraction in thyroid disease, exophthalmos (protruding eye), or enophthalmos (sunken eye). If the fissure is larger on one side, it gives the appearance of one eye looking larger than the other, but is almost never due to disparity in the size of the globe. One rare exception is an enlarged globe in congenital glaucoma (Fig. 6.104).

Blepharoptosis (also called ptosis)

Ptosis refers to a dropping lid with narrowing of the palpebral fissure. It may be present at birth in which case it is usually due to under-action of the levator m. and is followed without surgery if it is not obstructing vision. The most common reason for acquired ptosis is degeneration of the levator m. with aging or a partial traumatic disinsertion of the levator m. from the tarsal plate (Figs 4.26 and 4.27).

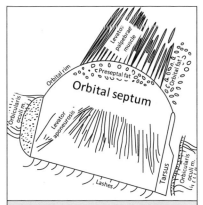

Fig. 4.26 The orbital septum thickens to form the tarsal plate (see Fig. 5.1). The levator palpebral m. originates in the orbital apex. Its aponeurosis then passes through and inserts onto the anterior tarsal plate. The orbicularis m. that closes the lids, overlies the levator m. and its fibers must be split to expose the levator m.

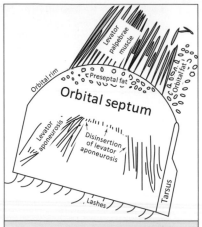

Fig. 4.27 Partial disinsertion of the levator palpebral aponeurosis from the tarsal plate.

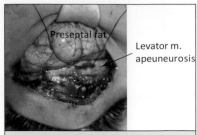

Fig. 4.28 Repair of ptosis by surgically advancing the levator palpebrae aponeurosis and suturing it to the inferior tarsus.

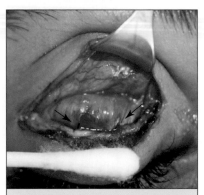

Fig. 4.29 Disinserted levator aponeurosis in previous figure sutured to inferior tarsus (Fig. 4.28). Courtesy of Joseph A. Mauriello, Jr., MD.

Surgical correction of the ptosis depends on the amount of levator m. function still present. With good levator m. action, an advancement of the muscle on the tarsal plate is sufficient (Figs 4.28 and 4.29). Sometimes, one must also resect a piece of the muscle which further tightens it. With little levator function, as in congenital ptosis, a frontalis sling operation is pervoformed where the tarsal plate is connected to the frontalis m. above the brow.

Periodically occurring ptosis by itself, or with diplopia, may be the first sign of myasthenia gravis. In this myoneural junction disorder, the ptosis may worsen when tired, or after a provocative test such as asking the patient to look up for several minutes (Figs 4.30 and 4.31).

Other neurologic causes of ptosis are CN III paralysis (Figs 4.30 and 4.31) sympathetic n. dysfunction (Figs 3.43 and 3.44).

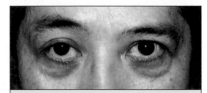

Fig. 4.30 Myasthenia gravis: no ptosis.

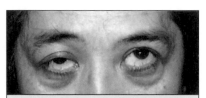

Fig. 4.31 Myasthenia gravis: ptosis after looking up for 5 minutes.

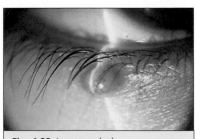

Fig. 4.32 Ingrown lash.

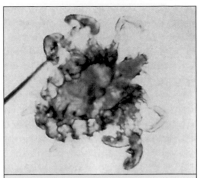

Fig. 4.33 Crab lice (*Phthirius pubis*) on lashes.

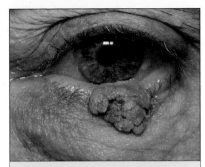

Fig. 4.34 Verruca vulqaris (wart) with its typical cauliflower-like appearance. Courtesy of Michael Stanley, Medical College of Georgia.

Lashes

Trichiasis (inturned lashes) (Figs 4.24 and 6.13) causes corneal irritations, and may be the result of an entropion (inturned lid), or trauma to the lid margin. Lashes can be epilated (pulled out), or the lash follicles can be destroyed with electrolysis or cryosurgery.

Lashes sometimes grow under the skin (Fig. 4.32) and may be removed after injection of local anesthetic.

Lice (pediculosis capitis) on the scalp hair, and lashes cause blepharitis and conjunctivitis (Fig. 4.33). There are 6 million cases a year in the US, mainly in children aged 3–12. Rx: Kwell shampoo.

Madarosis refers to loss of eyelashes and/or eyebrows. It may be due to skin disease, trauma, infection, and epilation due to psychiatric reasons (trichotillomania).

Verrucas (warts) (Fig. 4.34), caused by the papilloma virus, and molluscum contagiosum (Fig. 4.35), caused by the pox virus, are both common skin lesions of the lid. Either may cause conjunctivitis, especially when near the lid margin. Molluscum is usually treated with curettage of the central umbilicated dimple. The verruca is excised with cauterization of the base.

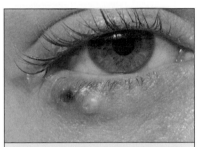

Fig. 4.35 Molluscum contagiosum are small, firm, rounded umbilicated papules with caseous material in the center. They may be single or multiple. Courtesy of Malcolm Luxemberg, MD and Arch of Ophth, Sept 1986, Vol 104, p. 1390. Copyright 1986, Amer, Med. Assoc. All rights reserved.

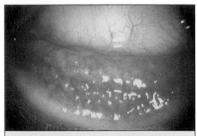

Fig. 4.36 Follicular conjunctivitis due to viral molluscum contagiosum. Courtesy of Malcolm Luxemberg, MD and Arch of Ophth, Sept 1986, Vol 104, p. 1390. Copyright 1986, Amer, Med. Assoc. All rights reserved.

Seborrheic keratosis (Fig. 4.37), which is common with aging, is a benign, brown, rough-surfaced growth appearing stuck on like clay thrown against a wall. It is excised for cosmetic reasons.

Epidermoid inclusion cysts (Fig. 4.38) are intracutaneous benign, smooth, glistening, white balls filled with cheesy substance and are excised for cosmetic reasons.

Nevi (Fig. 4.39) are benign, non-pigmented or pigmented, well-demarcated growths from early childhood. Suspect malignancy if there is: growth, irregular edges, inflammation, satellites, irregular pigment, ulceration, or bleeding.

Keratoacanthoma (Fig. 4.40) is a benign growth that resolves spontaneously. Rolled edges with umbilicated center filled with keratin make it difficult to distinguish from squamous carcinoma, so a biopsy is sometimes indicated.

Infantile hemangiomas (Fig. 4.41) are the most common, benign tumors of the lid and orbit in children. They appear shortly after birth, affecting 1–3% of infants, and often regress by 2–3 years of age. Treatment is necessary if it causes the lid to block vision or if it causes strabismus or compression of the globe. Systemic or intralesional corticosteroids are often the preferred regimen; but laser, surgical excision, and, most recently, systemic or topical beta blockers may be tried.

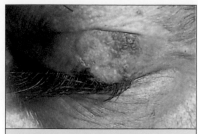
Fig. 4.37 Seborrheic keratosis.

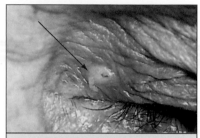
Fig. 4.38 Epidermoid inclusion cyst.

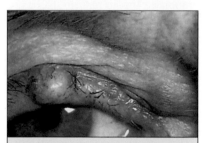
Fig. 4.39 Nevus.

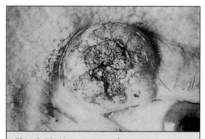
Fig. 4.40 Keratoacanthoma.

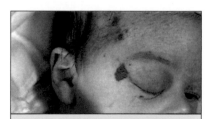
Fig. 4.41 Infantile hemangioma.

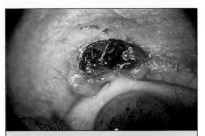

Fig. 4.42 Carcinoma of the lid is usually basal cell, but squamous cell looks similar and is also common.

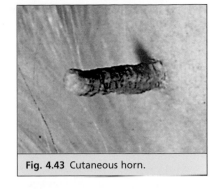

Fig. 4.43 Cutaneous horn.

The lids, face and scalp are the most common locations for basal cell carcinoma, and, less often, squamous cell carcinoma, of the skin (Fig. 4.42). They are strongly related to exposure to the sun's ultraviolet rays. Basal and squamous cell carcinomas are the most common malignancies in humans , occurring in 1 in 5 Americans. All chronic, hard, nodular, umbilicated, ulcerated, vascularized lesions demand a biopsy. Recommend that everyone, especially fair-skinned individuals avoid excessive exposure to the sun.

Cutaneous horns (Fig. 4.43) are keratinized overgrowths of seborrheic keratosis, verruca, or squamous or basal cell carcinoma; therefore, a biopsy of the base is indicated

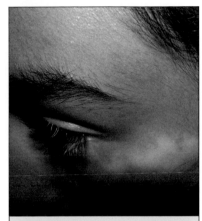

Fig. 4.44 Ash-leaf spots on the skin are multiple, depigmented macules with irregular borders. They are usually the first sign of tuberous sclerosis and appear in up to 90% of patients.

Phakomatoses

Congenital syndromes, which include lesions of the brain, skin, and eye are called phakomatoses. The early onset of skin lesions in these infants and young children provide a red flag to alert one to other problems.

1. Tuberous sclerosis is a condition appearing in the first 3 years of life consisting of seizures, mental deficiency, and sebaceous adenomas. Seventy-five percent of patients die before age 20 (Figs 4.44 and 4.45).

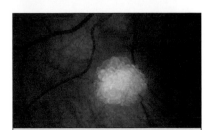

Fig. 4.45 Retinal astrocytoma in tuberous sclerosis. Areas of calcification give mulberry appearance. Courtesy of Dana Gabel Barnes Retinal Institute, St Louis, MO.

2. Sturge-Weber syndrome includes facial port wine capillary malformations (Fig. 4.46) and mental retardation in half of the patients. They should be monitored for early onset glaucoma and choroidal and CNS hemangiomas.

3. Neurofibromatosis is a condition that is inherited in an autosomal dominant pattern with incomplete penetrance. Tumors could affect the optic nerve, iris, retina, and skin of the lid (Fig. 4.47). Lisch nodules in the iris are present in 94% of patients (Fig. 4.48). Brown macular lesions occur early on and eventually in 99% of patients.

Leprosy is a chronic disease caused by acid-fast *Mycobacterium leprae*. It is probably transmitted by the respiratory route and usually involves prolonged exposure in childhood.

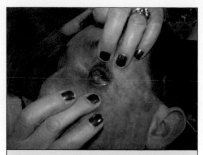

Fig. 4.46 Sturge–Weber syndrome.

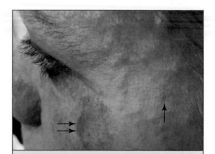

Fig. 4.47 Neurofibromatosis (von Recklinhausen disease) is characterized by neurofibromas of the skin (↑) and nervous system, and cafe-au-lait spots (↓↓), which are irregularly shaped brown macules. There are usually 5 or more, increasing in size from 0.5cm to 1.5cm in adults.

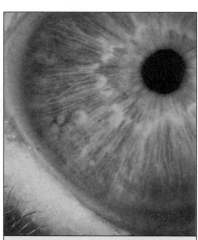

Fig. 4.48 Lisch nodules on the iris of a patient with neurofibromatosis. Courtesy of S. J. Charles, FRCS and *Arch. Ophth.*, Nov. 1989, Vol. 107, p. 1572. Copyright 1989, Amer. Med. Assoc. All rights reserved.

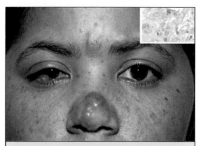

Fig. 4.49 Twenty-two year old from Cape Verde Islands with lepromatous leprosy. There are macular and erythematous nodular lesions on face, trunk, and extremities. Fite's stain/acid fast bacilli in skin biopsy confirms the diagnosis.

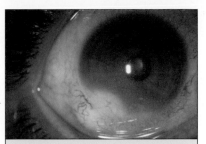

Fig. 4.50 Leprosy causing a solid nodule on the ocular surface together with granulomatous iritis. Courtesy of Carly Seidman, BS and Arch of Ophth., Dec 2010, Vol 128, p. 1522. Copyright 2010, Amer. Med. Assoc. All rights reserved.

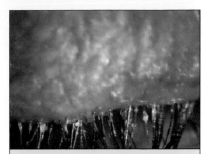

Fig. 4.51 Anterior blepharitis with crusting flakes on lashes. Courtesy of Michael Lemp, MD.

Anterior and posterior blepharitis

Blepharitis refers to inflammation or infection of the lid margin. It is extremely common and there is rarely a day that goes by that an eye doctor doesn't treat it or one of its sequelae, such as conjunctivitis, sties, chalazions, corneal ulcers, lid cellulitis, dry eye, or intolerance to contact lenses.

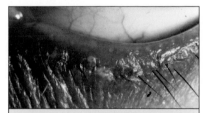

Fig. 4.52 Anterior blepharitis with crusting and ulcerative lesions around lashes. Courtesy of Michael Lemp, MD.

The anterior type manifests with crusting, redness, and ulcerative lesions around the lashes (Figs 4.51 and 4.52). It is often associated with scalp dandruff. The posterior type is due to infection of the meibomian glands. These glands normally secrete the oily meibum that helps minimize tear evaporation and lubricate the eye so as to minimize discomfort from the estimated 50,000 blinks per day. Many times, these glands become dysfunctional and produce a white, pasty secretion that predisposes the glands to infection (Figs 4.3 and 4.55). To minimize the incidence of infection, predisposed patients routinely cleanse the margin with baby shampoo or commercially available lid scrubs together with warm compresses which remove toxic debris and desquamated cells.

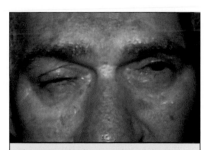

Fig. 4.53 Blepharoconjunctivitis in acne rosacea. This chronic condition is associated with engorged vessels and pustules on the nose, forehead, cheeks, and chin.

When infection does occur – usually due to staphylococcus – topical ophthalmic antibiotic

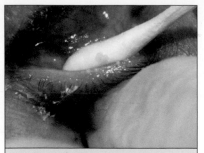

Fig. 4.54 Posterior blepharitis: dysfunctional meibomian glands are a common, chronic problem characterized by a toothpaste-like secretion. The glands are predisposed to infection causing posterior blepharitis and/or a chalazion.

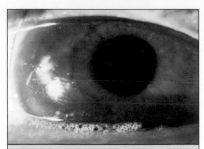

Fig. 4.55 Posterior blepharitis with foamy residue overlying the meibomian glands. This breakdown product of abnormal secretions may irritate the eye. Courtesy of Michael Lemp MD.

drops and/or ointments with or without steroids may be used, Generic tobramycin (Tobrex), polymyxin/trimethoprim (Polytrim) solution, and bacitracin ointment are highly effective. Generic tobramycin/dexamethasone (Tobradex) also reduces the inflammatory response to staphylococcus toxins and scaling debris. Oral generic doxycycline has antibacterial and anti-inflammatory effectiveness; but because of its systemic side effects, is reserved for more recalcitrant episodes. Squeezing the meibomian glands between a sterile cotton applicator and your finger tip, followed by placement of Betadine on the lid margins helps speed recovery (Fig. 4.54). This technique of eliciting discharge is also diagnostic when the diagnosis of posterior blepharitis is in doubt. Patients should be reminded that each episode of blepharitis could be treated, but it often recurs.

Chalazions (Fig. 4.57) are cystic enlargements of the meibomian glands that are due to clogging of an orifice. They could last for months. A chalazion is often incised and

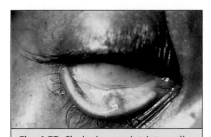

Fig. 4.56 Anterior and posterior blepharitis is often occur together and could cause sties and chalazions.

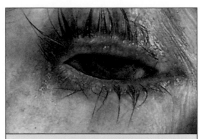

Fig. 4.57 Chalazions point internally.

drained (Fig. 4.58). If they become infected, antibiotic and/or steroid eye drops are added.

Sties are infections of the glands of Zeis and Moll around the lashes. These pimples are treated with hot soaks, local antibiotics, and incision. Systemic antibiotics are indicated if there is significant surrounding cellulitis.

Lid cellulitis is a diffuse infection often due to a sty, chalazion, bug bite, or cut. Lids are red and tender (Fig. 4.60). There may be adenopathy and fever. Rx: topical and systemic antibiotics. Shriveled skin, as in Fig. 4.19, is an initial indication that lid cellulitis is responding to treatment. Be cautious. When extensive, a CT scan could rule out involvement of sinuses or orbit.

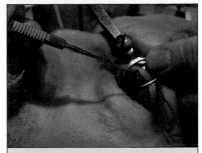

Fig. 4.58 A chalazion clamp is used to minimize bleeding during incision and curettage.

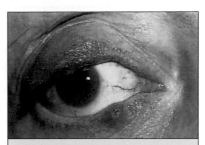

Fig. 4.59 Sties point externally.

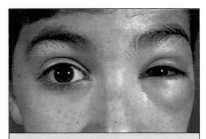

Fig. 4.60 Lid cellulitis.

Chapter 5

The orbit

The orbit is a cone-shaped vault (Figs 5.1 and 5.2). At its apex are three orifices through which pass the nerves, arteries, and veins supplying the eye.

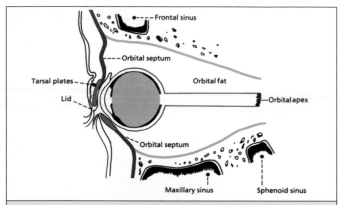

Fig. 5.1 Side view of orbit: periosteum (periorbita) of the orbit (green), the orbit septum (red) and tarsal plate (blue) are continuous connective tissue membranes. This fibrous membrane then goes on to cover the optic nerve as it exits the orbit and is then continuous with the dura mater covering the brain.

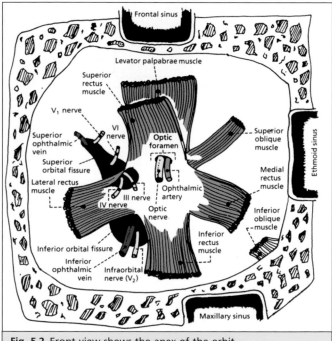

Fig. 5.2 Front view shows the apex of the orbit.

Unlike the eye in which most parts are amenable to direct visualization, evaluation of the orbit often requires the use of diagnosic tools such as CT scans and MRI.

Computed tomography (CT) scans are usually the radiologic technique of choice to evaluate orbital diseases such as fracture, foreign bodies, thyroid disease (Fig. 1.2) and sinusitis (Figs 5.3–5.5; 5.8).

CT scanning has made amazing contributions to medical diagnosis, but is a large contributor to the six-fold increase in diagnostic radiation in the last 30 years, because of overutilization. It is predicted that CT scans may be responsible for 1.5–2.0% of all future cancers in the US and studies reveal that patients are not informed of this risk 90–95% of the time.

Sinusitis

The orbit is surrounded on four sides by the paranasal sinuses, i.e., maxillary, frontal, sphenoid and ethmoid. Pain described as deep, or behind the eye, is most often due to allergy or infection of these sinuses. Pressure applied to the skin overlying the inflamed frontal, maxillary, and ethmoidal sinuses may cause tenderness (Fig. 5.3). The sphenoid sinus is behind the globe and cannot be tested in this way.

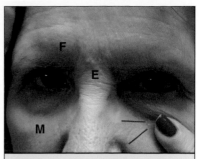

Fig. 5.3 One evidence of sinusitis is to elicit tenderness by palpating over the frontal (F), ethmoid (E), or maxillary (M) sinus. In this case the left maxillary sinus is involved.

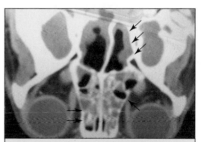

Fig. 5.4 CT scan showing three typical findings of ethmoiditis. A fluid level (↑) and opacification of the air spaces (↑↑) are common in an acute process. Thickening of mucosal membrane is more typical of chronicity (↑↑↑).

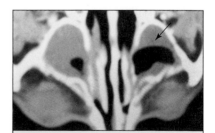

Fig. 5.5 CT scan of sphenoidal sinusitis with air-fluid level (↑).

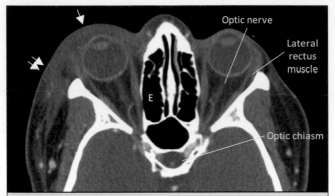

Optic nerve

Lateral rectus muscle

E

Optic chiasm

Fig. 5.6 CT scan showing preseptal lid swelling (↑) and periorbital cellulitis. The retrobulbar areas of the orbit and the ethmoid (E) sinuses are normal. There are, as yet, normal eye movements and no proptosis. Mild, early cases could be followed up cautiously on an outpatient basis. Courtesy of Sandip Basak, MD.

Clues that may indicate disease of the orbit

A. Proptosis (exophthalmos)—forward bulging of the eye.
B. Enophthalmos—sunken eye.
C. Swollen lids (sometimes totally shut); redness and engorgement of conjunctival vessels; clear fluid under conjunctiva (chemosis).
D. Loss of eye movement (ophthalmoplegia) due to involvement of cranial nerves III, IV, and VI or local damage to extraocular muscles.

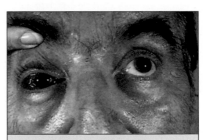

Fig. 5.7 Orbital cellulitis with chemosis and ophthalmoplegia, causing inability to look up.

Periorbital cellulitis causes swollen lids which may be totally shut (Figs 5.7 and 5.6). This may progress to the rarer and more serious orbital cellulitis (Fig. 5.8) in which the globe may not move (ophthalmoplegia) and there is chemosis, fever, adenopathy, and exophthalmos. It is due to sinusitis 60% of the time, but also occurs with tooth, facial, or lid infections.

A tough connective tissue called the periorbita lines the inner surface of the orbit. At the orbital rim, it becomes the orbital septum which then thickens to become the tarsal plate of the lid (see Fig. 5.1). This continuous fibrous membrane acts as a barrier protecting the orbit from lid and sinus infections and might be considered an 'orbital firewall'.

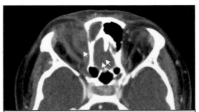

Fig. 5.8 CT scan of orbital cellulitis (↑) caused by ethmoid sinusitis (↑↑). Courtesy of Rand Kirtland, MD.

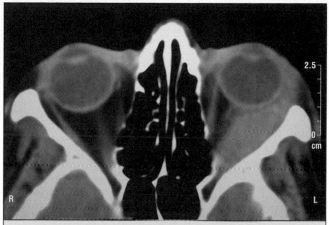

Fig. 5.9 MRI of left orbital pseudotumor, which is a non-infectious inflammation of the orbit. Courtesy of Egal Leibovich, MD and *Arch. Ophth.*, 2007, Vol. 125, No. 12, p. 1647–1651.

Beware of the rare breakthrough. If orbital cellulitis occurs, it can easily spread to the cavernous sinus through the superior and inferior ophthalmic veins that drain the orbit and part of the face. This could cause thrombosis and death. Hospitalize the patient and treat with systemic antibiotics.

Exophthalmos

Exophthalmos (proptosis) is a protrusion of the eyeball caused by an increase in orbital contents. It is measured with an exophthalmometer (Fig. 5.10). In adults, unilateral and bilateral cases are most often due to thyroid disease. In children, unilateral cases are most often due to orbital cellulitis. Other causes are metastatic tumors, orbital hemorrhage, cavernous sinus thrombosis or fistulas, sinus mucoceles, or the following primary orbital tumors:

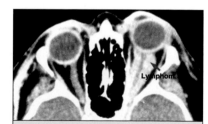

Fig. 5.10 Exophthalmometer.

1 hemangioma;
2 rhabdomyosarcoma;
3 pseudotumor (Fig. 5.9);
4 lipoma;
5 dermoid;
6 lacrimal gland tumor (Fig. 6.131);
7 glioma of the optic nerve;
8 lymphoma (Fig. 5.11);
9 meningioma.

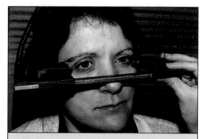

Fig. 5.11 CT scan of orbital lymphoma. Courtesy of Pfizer Pharmaceuticals.

Enophthalmos

Enophthalmos is a retracted globe. The most common cause is a blow to the orbit that raises intraorbital pressure, causing the thin roof of the maxillary sinus to fracture (Fig. 5.12). This is called a "blow-out" fracture. Associated signs may include subconjunctival hemorrhage, entrapment of the inferior rectus muscle in the fracture causing restriction of upward gaze, and vertical diplopia (Fig. 5.13). Decreased sensation (hypesthesia) of the cheek is due to infraorbital nerve damage (Fig. 5.14). If diplopia or enophthalmos persists; or if more than 50% of the floor is blown out; a silicone, polyethylene or titanium mesh may be inserted.

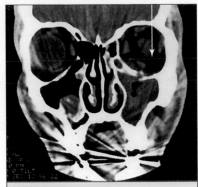

Fig. 5.12 Computed tomography (CT) scan of orbital blow-out fracture (↓).

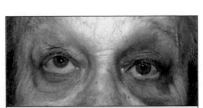

Fig. 5.13 Restriction of upward gaze due to blow-out fracture.

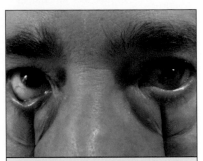

Fig. 5.14 Test for hypesthesia using 2 paper clips to compare the sensitivity on each side.

Chapter 6
Slit lamp examination and glaucoma

The slit lamp projects a beam of light onto the eye, which is viewed through a microscope (Fig. 6.1). The long wide beam is useful in scanning surfaces such as lids, conjunctiva, and sclera. The short narrow beam is used to study fine details (Figs 6.2 and 6.3).

Cornea

The cornea is the transparent, anterior continuation of the sclera devoid of both blood and lymphatic vessels. The grey corneal–scleral junction is called the limbus. A slit beam cross section of a normal cornea reveals the following, as shown in Figs 6.4 and 6.5:

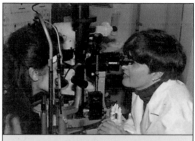

Fig. 6.1 Slit lamp.

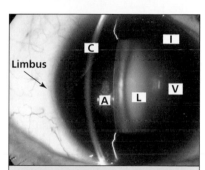

Fig. 6.3 Slit lamp view of anterior segment. (C, cornea; A, anterior chamber; I, iris; L, lens; V, vitreous). Courtesy of Takashi Fujikado, MD.

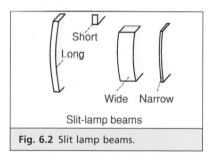

Short
Long
Wide Narrow
Slit-lamp beams

Fig. 6.2 Slit lamp beams.

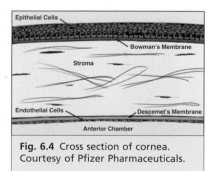

Epithelial Cells
Bowman's Membrane
Stroma
Endothelial Cells
Descemet's Membrane
Anterior Chamber

Fig. 6.4 Cross section of cornea. Courtesy of Pfizer Pharmaceuticals.

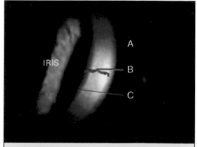

Fig. 6.5 Slit beam cross section of a cornea. A = epithelium, B = stroma, C = endothelium.

Manual for Eye Examination and Diagnosis, Eighth edition. Mark Leitman.
© 2012 John Wiley & Sons, Ltd. Published 2012 by John Wiley & Sons, Ltd.

1 anterior band: epithelium on Bowman's membrane;
2 cross section: through stroma;
3 posterior band: endothelium on Descemet's membrane.

The corneal epithelium is the superficial multilayered covering of the cornea that sits on Bowman's membrane (BM). Its cells regenerate quickly so that 40% of the surface could regenerate in 24 hours. New cells are generated in the deepest layer sitting on BM and move toward the surface. The epithelial cells are also formed from the embryonic stem cells in the limbus that migrate across the cornea.

The central stroma is the clear connective tissue layer containing the most densely packed number of sensory fibers in the body. Abrasions and inflammations (keratitis) are, therefore, very painfuL "Kerato" is a prefix that refers to cornea.

The deepest endothelial layer sits on Descemet's membrane and is only one cell thick and doesn't regenerate. Its function is to pump fluid out of the cornea to maintain clarity.

Corneal epithelial disease

Commonly occurring epithelial abrasions (Figs 6.6 and 6.7) due to trauma present with pain and a "red" eye. The de-epithelialized area stains bright green with fluorescein and a cobalt blue light. Rx: topical antibiotic, a cycloplegic (Cyclogel 1%), an oral analgesic, with a pressure patch (two patches). Most abrasions clear within 24–48 hours.

To facilitate the examination of painful eyes, anesthetize with topical proparacaine 0.5%. It acts in seconds and lasts a few minutes. Never prescribe it for relief of pain since continued use damages the cornea.

Rarely, chemical or surgical trauma to the surface is so severe it destroys a large area of the limbus. In these cases, the epithelium cannot regenerate properly and a cell transplant has to be done. Normal limbal tissue from the

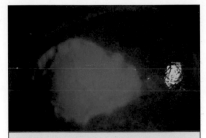

Fig. 6.6 Corneal abrasion. stained with fluorescein.

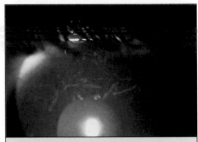

Fig. 6.7 Linear abrasions from trichiasis or particle under lid.

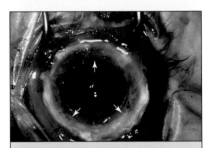

Fig. 6.8 360° limbal stem cell allograft: Sutured and glued to sclera (↑). Courtesy of Clara Chan, MD and Edward J. Holland, MD. Cincinnati Eye Institute.

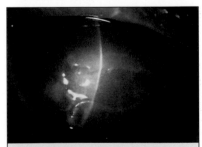

Fig. 6.9 Recurrent corneal erosion with localized epithelial edema.

patient's other eye (autograft), from a relative (allograft, Fig. 6.8) or a cadaver may be used.

Corneal foreign bodies are removed with a sterile needle after placing two drops of proparacaine. Antibiotic drops are then prescribed.

Localized epithelial edema (Fig. 6.9) has a translucent appearance, unlike an ulcer, which is opaque. In the common condition, called recurrent corneal erosion, a small patch of edema develops where the epithelium does not adhere well to Bowman's membrane. This often follows injury, but may be spontaneous. Patients awake in the morning with pain when cells slough off, usually just below the center of the cornea. The abrasion is treated with a patch and an antibiotic. The edematous epithelium is treated with hypertonic 2% or 5% sodium chloride solution (Muro 128) in the daytime and sodium chloride 5% ophthalmic ointment (Muro 128 ointment) at bedtime. If sloughing continues, roughing up Bowman's membrane with a needle (stromal puncture) increases adhesiveness of cells.

Superficial punctate keratitis (SPK) (Fig. 6.10) is epithelial edema, which appears as punctate hazy areas that stain with fluorescein, (Fig. 6.11). Burning, pain, and conjunctival redness may result.

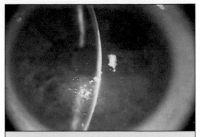

Fig. 6.10 Superficial punctate keratitis (SPK).

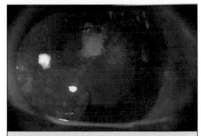

Fig. 6.11 Superficial punctate keratitis (SPK) stained with fluorescein.

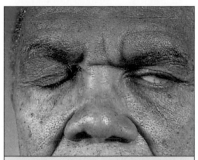

Fig. 6.12 Lagophthalmos is a condition in which the lids don't close completely.

Superficial punctate keratitis	
TRAUMATIC CAUSES	**DESSICATION**
• Contact lenses	• Dry eye due to decreased tear film production (p. 48)
• Ultraviolet light	
• Snow blindness	• Dry eye resulting from increased evaporation as results from:
• Reaction from eye drops	
• Chemical injury	1. Inability to close lids after over-correction following blepharoplasty
• Blepharitis	
• Trichiasis (Fig. 6.13)	2. VII N. paralysis (Bell's Palsy)
• Rubbing eyes	3. Thyroid exophthalmos

Corneal vascularization is a response to injury. Superficial vessels are most commonly a response to poorly fitting contact lenses (Fig. 6.14) but also grow into areas damaged from ulcers, lacerations, or chemicals.

Chemical injuries with basic substances, such as lye, are most ominous since they immediately penetrate the depths of the cornea and permanently scar (Figs 6.15 and 6.16). Acid burns usually do not penetrate stroma or scar. Rx: irrigate all chemical injuries immediately and profusely.

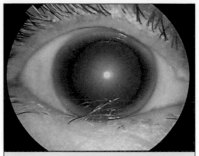

Fig. 6.13 Superficial punctate keratitis (SPK) from trichiasis.

Epidemic keratoconjunctivitis (Fig. 6.17) is a common, highly infectious condition due to one of the adenoviruses that cause the common cold. There may be a severe conjunctivitis lasting up to 3 weeks associated with photophobia, fever, cold symptoms, and an adenopathy. The main problem is the keratitis, which can last for months, and, rarely, years. It does not scar, but does restrict use of contact lenses until it clears. Wash your hands, instruments, chair and door knobs especially well after evaluating this eye infection.

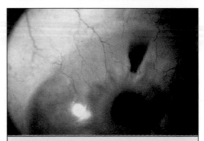

Fig. 6.14 Superficial vascularization often due to poorly fitting contact lenses. Courtesy of Michael Kelly.

Herpes simplex virus type 1 (HSV-l) is very common on the face especially around the eyes and lips. At age 4, about 25% of the population are seropositive and this approaches 100% by age 60. When the corneal epithelium (Figs 6.18 and 6.19) is involved, the lesions, called dendrites, are similar in appearance to a branching tree, especially when stained with fluorescein. Diffuse punctate or round lesions can also occur. Patients

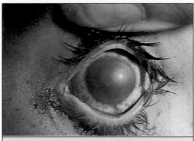

Fig. 6.15 Sodium hydroxide injury minutes later.

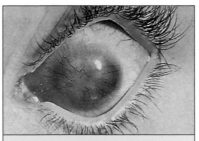

Fig. 6.16 Sodium hydroxide injury 3 months later.

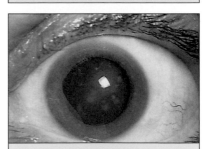

Fig. 6.17 Epidemic keratoconjunctivitis with characteristic white punctate subepithelial infiltrates.

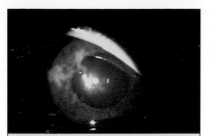

Fig. 6.18 Herpes simplex keratitis with tree-like branching lesions without fluorescein.

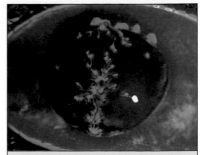

Fig. 6.19 Herpes simplex with large fluorescein stained dendrites. Courtesy of Allan Connor, Princess Margaret Hospital, Toronto, Canada.

complain of a gritty ocular sensation, conjunctivitis, and an occasional fever sore on the lip, nose, or mouth. There may be small vesicles on the skin of the lids (Fig. 6.20). These often crust and then disappear within three weeks. It should be treated quickly since it could cause corneal opacities and loss of vision. When it penetrates the stroma, a chronic keratitis and iritis will require the cautious addition of topical steroids. Recurrences are common. Rx: generic trifluridine (Viroptic) 1% every two hours has been the mainstay treatment for years, but newly introduced Zirgan gel can be used q3h and is less toxic. Valtrex 500 mg PO BID for 5 days may be added in resistant cases.

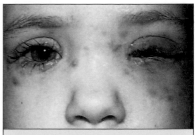

Fig. 6.20 Herpes dermatitis.

Anxious patients must be reassured that this eye disease is rarely due to HSV-2, which is a venereal disease transmitted by sexual contact.

Corneal ulcers are infections that are usually due to a bacterial, but occasionally to a viral and rarely a fungal infection. They are characterized by conjunctivitis and a white patch of inflammatory cells in the cornea. Over 50% result from contact lens wear, especially lenses worn during sleep. Other causes include corneal abrasions, conjunctivitis and blepharitis. Treat vigorously on an emergency basis, since it almost always scars and, in the case of *Pseudomonas*, may perforate within one day (Fig. 6.23).

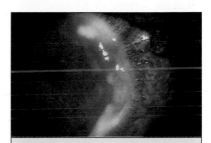

Fig. 6.21 Marginal corneal ulceration.

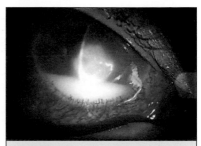

Fig. 6.22 Central corneal ulcer with secondary hypopyon.

Marginal ulcers (Fig. 6.21) are most common and may be due to infection or an immune reaction to staphylococcal toxins from associated chronic blepharitis. Rx: topical hourly broad-spectrum antibiotics. Steroids are sometimes added with caution.

Central ulcers (Fig. 6.22) are most ominous and in these cases, cultures are always needed. Topical broad-spectrum antibiotics are used up to every 15 minutes.

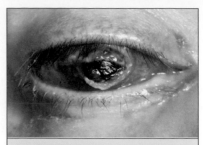

Fig. 6.23 Perforated corneal ulcer. Courtesy of Elliot Davidoff, MD.

The infection infrequently enters the globe (Fig. 6.22). When it does, a level of white cells may be seen in the anterior chamber, which is the space bounded anteriorly by the cornea and posteriorly by the iris and lens. This is called a hypopyon and might require a culture of the interior eye, especially if the vitreous is also involved.

Corneal endothelial disease

A monolayer of endothelial cells covers the deepest layer of the cornea and pumps fluid from the stroma to maintain corneal clarity. There are usually 2,800 endothelial cells/mm² which do not replicate. When the number of cells drops below 500, or are damaged, corneal edema can occur and blurry vision and discomfort may result (Figs 6.24–6.26). The most common cause for this edema is cataract surgery. In these cases, the endothelial cells may be injured mechanically, chemically, or from rejection of the lens implant. This complication of cataract surgery

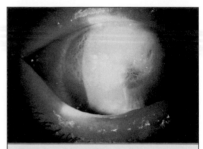

Fig. 6.24 Severe corneal edema with epithelial cysts is referred to as bullous keratopathy. It reduces vision and is usually very uncomfortable often breaking down to painful corneal abrasions. Courtesy of Kenneth R. Kenyon, MD and *Arch. Ophth.*, Mar. 1976, Vol. 94, p. 499–95. Copyright, 1976, Amer. Med. Assoc. All rights reserved.

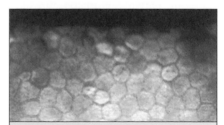

Fig. 6.26 Specular microscopy after cataract surgery that damaged the endothelium and caused corneal edema resulting in a cell count of 680 cells/mm². If cells are damaged they do not multiply to fill the gap. Instead, they enlarge and lose their normal hexagonal shape and their ability to pump fluid from the cornea. Courtesy of Martin Schneider, MD.

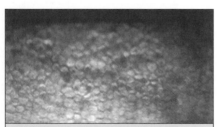

Fig. 6.25 Specular microscopy of normal endothelial cell count 2600 cells/mm² before cataract surgery.

is the most common reason for needing corneal transplant surgery. Elevated intraocular pressure (Fig. 6.103), iritis, and a genetic weakness of the endothelium in Fuch's dystrophy (Fig. 6.28) are also common causes. Very high pressure, often over 40 mmHg in acute angle-closure glaucoma (Figs 6.96, 6.97 and 6.125), temporarily damages the endothelium and causes corneal edema with the classic symptom of halos around lights. Symmetrel (amantadine), used to treat Parkinson's disease, could cause corneal edema by decreasing the endothelial cell count. Low pressure, below 5 mmHg, could also cause corneal cloudiness (Fig. 6.27).

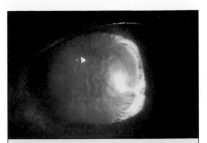

Fig. 6.27 Edematous folds in the cornea—called stria—usually result from low intracular pressure. It is a similar effect to a balloon not fully blown up.

Fuch's dystrophy is a genetic disorder of the Descemet's endothelial complex (Fig. 6.28) that results in drop out of endothelial cells. It is bilateral and is identified by guttata which are small round spots of thickening in Descemet's membrane. They are usually in the central corneal axis. It could lead to corneal edema and eventually require corneal transplant surgery.

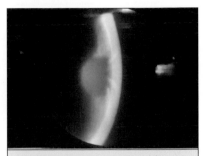

Fig. 6.28 Fuch's dystrophy with central comeal thickening and haze due to edema. Courtesy of Hank Perry, MD.

Corneal transplantation (keratoplasty)

Keratoplasty is one of the most successful organ transplant surgeries with more than a 90% success-rate at one year and 80% after 10 years. In 2009, 23,000 full-thickness penetrating keratoplasties (PK) (Figs 6.29 and 6.30) and 18,000 Descemet's stripping endothelial keratoplasties (DSEK) (Figs 6.31–6.34) were performed in the US using donor corneas from eyebanks. PK is used to replace scarred opacified stroma and sometimes to replace damaged endothelium. Two problems with PK is that it requires extensive suturing, which remains in place for over a year and could take that amount of time for visual return. Also, there is often a lot of residual astigmatism. In DSEK, just the diseased endothelium and Descemet's membrane are replaced through a small wound resulting in earlier return of vision. A third type of keratoplasty, called

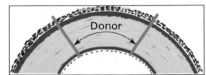

Fig. 6.29 Full-thickness corneal transplant (PK).

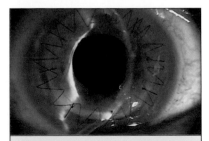

Fig. 6.30 Full thickness corneal transplant (penetrating keratopathy).

deep anterior lamellar keraplasty (DALK) is done less frequently (1,000/year) (Figs 6.35–6.39). In DALK, just the anterior cornea is replaced leaving behind the endothelium and Descemet's membrane. Its advantage is that the patient's endothelial cells usually have a longer survival rate than the donor's. Immunologic endothelial cell rejection is the leading cause of corneal graft failure.

A human corneal donor graft may be repeatedly rejected for immune reasons or because of a poor surface environment as with dry eye or with a vascularized cornea as occurs with chemical burns (Figs 6.15 and 6.16). A

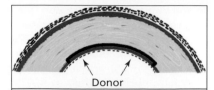

Fig. 6.31 DSEK: After removing damaged endothelium and Descemet's membrane, the donor tissue is folded to fit through a small wound. An air bubble is injected to press the donor graft against the cornea. The endothelial cells, natural pumping action hold the graft in place without sutures.

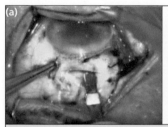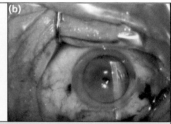

Fig. 6.32 Replacement of endothelium and Descemet's membrane. (a) Stripping of 8.0 mm diameter of diseased endothelium and Descemet's membrane. (b) Insertion of folded donor graft. Reproduced from *Br. J. Ophthalmol.*, July 2010, Vol 94, No. 7, Studeny et al. Copyright BMJ Publishing Group Ltd.

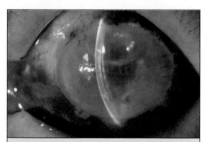

Fig. 6.33 DSEK graft separation (↑) three days after transplant. It was reattached by injecting an air bubble. Courtesy of Christopher Rapuano, MD, Chief, Cornea Service, Wills Eye Hospital.

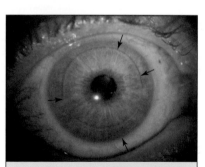

Fig. 6.34 Successful DSEK surgery with implant in place (↑). Courtesy of Henry Perry, MD.

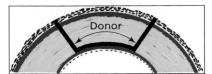

Fig. 6.35 Deep anterior lamellar keratoplasty (DALK) removes all the stroma up to Descemet's membrane. A common complication is penetration of this thin, 10mm layer. This necessitates converting to a penetrating keratoplasty 20% of the time.

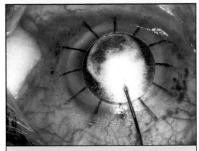

Fig. 6.36 DALK: Step 1 is to inject air into the corneal stroma to begin separation of stroma from Descemet's membrane.

last effort at maintaining clarity in the central axis is implantation of a graft utilizing a centrally located plastic lens (Figs 6.40 and 6.41). In 2007, 639 grafts, Boston type, were done. A complication unique to this keratoplasty procedure is retroprosthetic membranes.

Keratoconus (Figs 6.42 and 6.43) is a bilateral central thinning and bulging (ectasia) of the cornea to a conical shape. It is due to weakening of the stromal collagen. It begins between ages 10 and 30, often in allergic persons and in patients with Down's syndrome. There is a higher incidence within families.

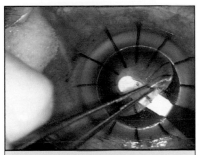

Fig. 6.37 Step 2 is to complete stromal dissection with crescent blade.

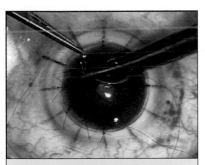

Fig. 6.39 Step 4 is to suture donor graft to recipient bed. Reprinted from *Am. J. Ophthal.* Vol. 148/5. Daphne C.Y. Han, Jodhbir S. Mehta, Yang Ming Por, Hla Myint Htoon, Donald T.H. Tan. Comparison of Outcomes of Lamellar Keratoplasty and Penetrating Keratoplasty in Keratoconus, Nov. 2009, with permission from Elsevier.

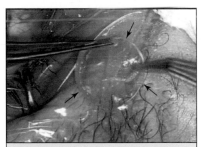

Fig. 6.38 Step 3 is to remove Descemet's membrane from the donor cornea (↑).

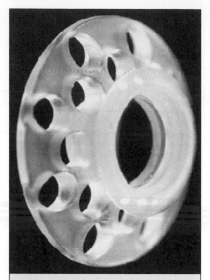

Fig. 6.40 The Boston Keratoprosthesis – collar-button device made of PMMA plastic. It is incorporated into a corneal graft that serves as carrier which is sutured in place like a standard graft.

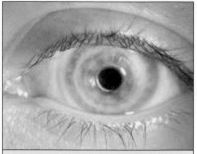

Fig. 6.41 Eye of a 23 year-old patient with congenital endothelial dystrophy. Four standard corneal grafts had failed. A Boston Keratoprosthesis implanted 5 years earlier resulted in consistent vision of 20/30, and normal pressure. Courtesy of Claes Dohlman, MD, PhD.

The resulting irregular type of astigmatism corrects poorly with glasses and may need contact lenses to obtain clearer vision.

If the cornea continues to steepen, one may try to flatten it with intrastromal rings (Fig. 2.51) or chemically strengthen the stromal collagen with a new technique called cross-linking. In this procedure, riboflavin 0.1% solution is continuously dropped into the cornea while the eye is irradiated with UV light for 1/2 hour. It should only be used in cases of documented progression of disease.

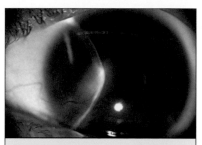

Fig. 6.42 Keratoconus.

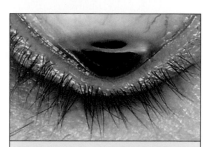

Fig. 6.43 Munson's sign: conical cornea indents lid when looking down. Courtesy of Michael P. Kelly.

Down's syndrome occurs in about 1:800 births and is due to trisomy of chromosome 21. It is characterized by mental retardation, short stature, and a transverse palmar crease ("simian crease"). Besides keratoconus, there is an increased incidence of strabismus, cataracts, and refractive errors. (Fig. 6.44).

Argyrosis results from long-term exposure to topical or systemic silver (Fig. 6.45a). Silver nitrate 2% eyedrops was used extensively as anti-infective in the first half of the 20th century. It was the mainstay prophylactic therapy in newborns.

Wilson's disease (hepatolenticular degeneration) is characterized by excessive deposition of copper in the liver and brain. It is a rare autosomal recessive disorder that often begins before age 40. The plasma copper-carrying protein—serum ceruplasmin—is low. The pathognomonic sign of the condition is the brownish or grey-green Kayser-Fleischer ring (Fig. 6.45b) due to copper deposits in Descemet's membrane, adjacent to the limbus.

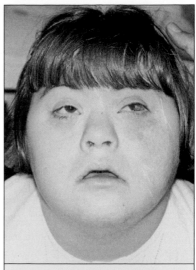

Fig. 6.44 Down's Syndrome patient with keratoconus. Corneal edema (hydrops) is caused by a tear in Descemet's membrane. Also, note the characteristic flat face, small nose, low nasal bridge, narrow interpupillary distance, and upward slanting palpebral fissures. Courtesy of Kenneth R. Kenyon, MD and *Arch. Ophth.*, Mar. 1976, Vol. 94, p. 494–495, Copyright 1976, Amer. Med. Assoc., All rights reserved.

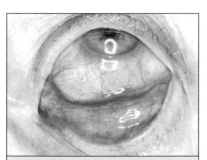

Fig. 6.45a Argyrosis: Deposition of silver in conjunctiva, cornea and lid. Silver nitrate eyedrops were used in the past as a prophylactic anti-bacterial in newborns. Courtesy of Elliot Davidoff, MD.

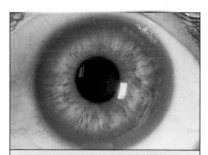

Fig. 6.45b Copper deposited in Descemet's membrane causing an orange ring at the limbus is pathognomonic of Wilson's disease. Compare with corneal arcus shown in Appendix 2.8. Courtesy of Denise de Freitas, MD. Paulista School of Medicine, Sao Paulo, Brazil.

Dermoid tumors (Fig. 6.46) are benign congenital growths often having protruding hairs. They are most common at the corneal limbus or in the orbit and may grow during puberty. They are removed if vision is threatened or for cosmetic reasons.

Conjunctiva

The conjunctiva is a mucous membrane. The bulbar conjunctiva covers the sclera and ends at the corneal limbus. The palpebral conjunctiva lines the lids (Fig. 6.47). Fluid within the conjunctiva is called chemosis (Fig. 6.48) and is commonly seen in allergy and in rare cases of orbital venous congestion.

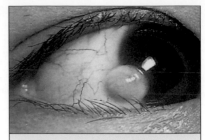

Fig. 6.46 Corneal dermoid.

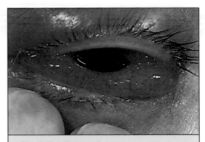

Fig. 6.48 Chemosis.

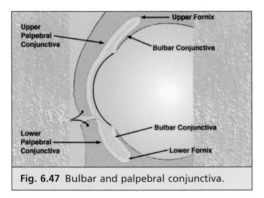

Fig. 6.47 Bulbar and palpebral conjunctiva.

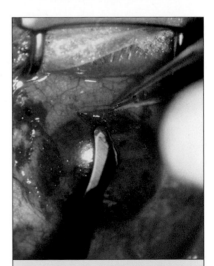

Fig. 6.49b A pterygium is removed with a superficial lamellar dissection and excision of adjacent paralimbal conjunctiva. An autograft of conjunctiva from another area of the same eye is sutured to adjacent paralimbal area to reduce recurrences of the pterygium. Frua E, et al. *Acta Ophthalmol. Scand.* 2004.

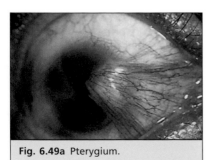

Fig. 6.49a Pterygium.

To examine the inner surface of the upper lid, first warn the patient, then "flip the lid" as follows:

1 have the patient look down with eyes open;
2 grasp eyelashes of upper lid at their bases;
3 pull out and up on lashes while pushing in and down on upper tarsal margin (patient should continue to look down during examination);
4 to return lid to normal position, have the patient look up.

A pterygium (Fig. 6.49a, b) is a triangular growth of vascularized conjunctiva encroaching on the nasal cornea. Two causes are wind and ultraviolet light. It may be excised for cosmetic, comfort, or visual reasons. Recurrences of up to 30–40% are reported.

A pinguecula (Fig. 6.50) is a common, benign, yellowish elevation of the 180° conjunctiva, usually nasal but also temporal. It is composed of collagen and elastic tissue. It occasionally becomes red, especially with allergies (Fig. 6.51), and, rarely, may be removed if it is chronically inflamed, if it interferes with contact lens wear, or if it is a cosmetic problem.

Subconjunctival hemorrhages (Fig. 6.52) may be spontaneous, or result from rubbing of the eye, vomiting, coughing, elevated blood pressure, or, rarely, bleeding disorders. Recommend no rubbing, and no bearing down.

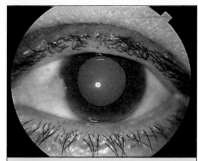

Fig. 6.50 Pinguecula.

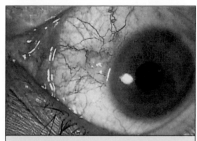

Fig. 6.51 Inflamed pinguecula.

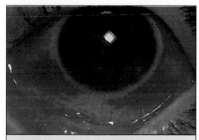

Fig. 6.52 Subconjunctival hemorrhage.

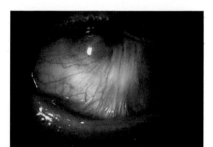

Fig. 6.53a Symblepharon: Adhesions of bulbar to palpebral conjunctiva should be lysed with a glass rod or wet cotton applicator to prevent permanent scar. From Kheirkhah et al., 2008, *Amer. J. Ophth.*, 146, p. 271. With permission from Elsevier.

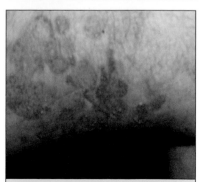

Fig. 6.53b Bullous pemphigoid causes conjunctivitis and itchy, red blisters on the skin.

A symblepharon (Figs 1.9 and 6.53a) is an adhesion of the bulbar and palpebral conjunctiva. Contracture can lead to an entropion with trichiasis. It is most commonly due to chemical burns, trachoma, epidemic keratoconjunctivitis and two immune blistering mucocutaneous diseases that involve the eye.

1. Stevens-Johnson syndrome, which is an immune reaction to a foreign antigen, usually a drug (Fig. 1.9), and could be fatal.

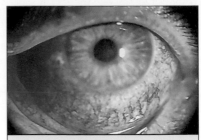
Fig. 6.54 Conjunctivitis.

2. Bullous pemphigoid (Fig. 6.53b) is an autoimmune condition involving the skin and conjunctiva. It could last for years, and unlike Stevens-Johnson, it is not fatal. It is also confirmed by biopsy. Pemphix is Latin for blister.

Conjunctivitis causes redness with a gritty sensation. Common causes are tired eyes, pollutants, wind, dust, dryness, allergy, or infection (Fig. 6.54). If there is pain, it usually indicates corneal or intraocular involvement. Vascularized elevations of the palpebral conjunctiva, called papillae (Fig. 6.55), are a reaction to an inflamed eye. It is most unique to giant papillary conjunctivitis and vernal conjunctivitis.

Giant papillary conjunctivitis (GPC) is a common cause for rejecting soft contact lenses. Large papillae develop are under the lids. They could which are an immune reaction usually to mucous debris on the lenses. Rx: change to a soft contact lens that is disposed of more frequently, i.e., every two weeks or even on a daily schedule; decrease wearing time; and keep lenses especially clean.

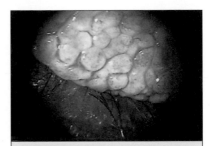
Fig. 6.55 Papillae of the palpebral conjunctiva.

Vernal conjunctivitis is an allergic condition in which large papillae are under the upper lid. They could abrade the cornea. It occurs in the first decade and may last for years. Both GPC and vernal conjunctivitis may be treated with a topical mast-cell inhibitor such as Cromolyn 4% solution and less often with steroid drugs.

White lymphoid elevations of the conjunctiva (Fig. 6.56) called follicles occur as a reaction to conjunctival irritation, especially from viruses, *Chlamydia*, and drugs.

1 Trachoma is a severe keratoconjunctivitis due to an infection by *Chlamydia trachomatis*. It affects 146 million people worldwide and is

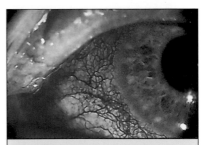
Fig. 6.56 Follicles of the palpebral conjunctiva.

responsible for blindness in 6 million people outside the USA. It begins with papillae and follicles on the superior palpebral conjunctiva. Conjunctival shortening may result in an entropion, which causes trichiasis. Inflammation of the cornea leads to superior vascularization (pannus), occasional corneal scarring, and loss of vision (Fig. 6.57). Rx: a single dose of azithromycin, 20 mg/kg.

2 Inclusion conjunctivitis in adults is a follicular conjunctivitis with occasional keratitis. It is also due to *Chlamydia trachomatis* of a different serotype than that causing trachoma. This organism is the most common sexually transmitted pathogen—and, therefore, must be ruled out in sexually active people. It is the most common cause of conjunctivitis in newborns, who acquire it passing through the birth canal. Confirm with smear or culture. Rx: oral doxycycline, tetracycline, or azithromycin, and erythromycin ophthalmic ointment; treat sexual partners.

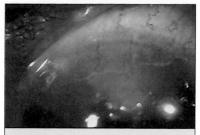

Fig. 6.57 Corneal inflammation from trachoma.

Bacterial conjunctivitis has a white–yellow discharge and is often due to *Staphylococcus aureus*, *Streptococcus pneumoniae*, and *Haemophilus influenzae*. It is usually treated without cultures (Figs 6.58 and 6.59).

Inexpensive generic eye drops are used to treat simple infections of the conjunctiva and lids. Examples are gentamycin+, tobramycin^A, sulfacetamide*, and fluoroquinolones such as ofloxacin and ciprofloxacin* (*also comes in ointments). Popular combination drops are bacitracin/neomycin/polymyxin, and polymyxin/trimethoprim (Polytrim). Ointments blur vision and are most useful for bedtime use, especially on the lid margins. Two antibiotics available only as ointments are bacitracin and erythromycin. The latter is placed in the eyes of most newborns to prevent chlamydial and other causes of conjunctivitis which might be picked up passing through birth canal (Fig. 6.45a).

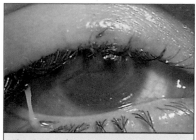

Fig. 6.58 Infectious conjunctivitis.

Chronic bacterial conjunctivitis, sties, chalazions, and blepharitis commonly occur in acne rosacea (Fig. 4.53). This erythematous pustular dermatitis affects the forehead, cheeks, chin, and nose. Telangiectatic vessels, especially on the nose, are pathognomonic.

Viruses cause half the infectious cases of conjunctivitis. There is usually a watery discharge associated with "cold symptoms" and a swollen preauricular node. It is often treated with antibiotics since it is difficult to be sure the infection is not bacterial and cultures are not usually practical. Antibiotic–steroid combinations, such as Tobradex, may relieve symptoms, but could aggravate an atypical herpes simplex infection.

Allergic conjunctivitis is a condition associated with itching, slight conjunctival injection, stringy mucous discharge, chemosis, and puffy lids. Treatment begins with avoidance of known irritants, discontinuing make-up, and applying cold compresses. When drops are needed, begin with over-the-counter (OTC) and then generic prescriptions, since they are less expensive and very effective. Ex. of OTC: Decongestants $7.00; decongestant/antihistamine $8.00; antihistamine/mast cell stabilizer $13.00. Prescription drops range from $40.00 to $100.00.

Naphcon A, Opcon A, and Visine A, available OTC, contain a combination of an antihistamine/vasoconstrictor (pheniramine maleate/naphazoline). They relieve discomfort and redness. The market cliché "GET THE RED OUT" is true, but has the negative effect of causing rebound hyperemia in the long run. These drugs also dilate the pupil and could rarely cause an attack of angle closure glaucoma. Caution the patient to call an eye doctor if they experience eye pain, blurry vision, or increased redness. Ketotifen (Zaditor or Alaway) is one of a group of OTC drugs that have antihistamine, mast cell stabilizer and eosinophil inhibitor actions with few side effects and is, therefore, safer for long-term use. Prescribe one drop twice a day. After trying antihistamines, decongestants, or mast cell stabilizers, non-steroid (NSAID), and then steroid, anti-inflammatories can be added or used alone. Generic Acular (ketorolac NSAID) drops may be prescribed QID prn. If symptoms

Conjunctivitis

	Viral	Bacterial	Allergic
Onset	Acute	Acute	Intermittent
Associated complaints	Often sore throat, rhinitis, fever	Often none	History of allergy; nasal or sinus stuffiness, dermatitis
Discharge	Watery	Thick, yellow	Stringy mucus
Preauricular node	Common	Nonpurulent	None

still persist, a steroid such as generic FML (fluorometholone) may be prescribed.

When steroids are used, the patient should be monitored by an eye doctor since they could elevate eye pressure or precipitate a herpes simplex infection.

Conjunctival nevi (Fig. 6.60) are common. Malignant transformation of nevi to melanomas is rare. Malignant transformation is suggested by satellites, rapid growth, elevation, and inflammation (Fig. 6.61) and occurs 75% of the time from a pre existing benign pigmented lesion.

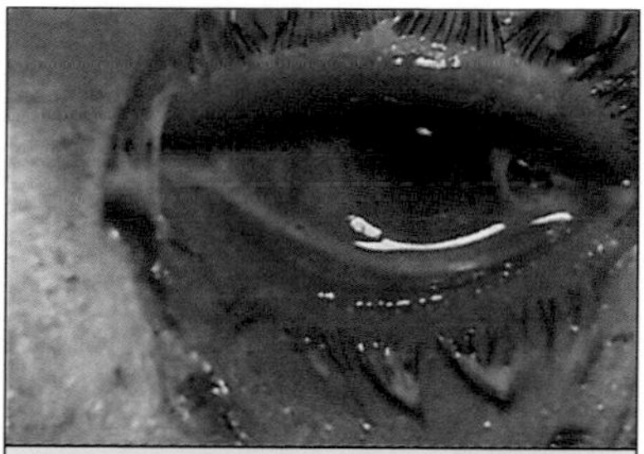

Fig. 6.59 Bacterial blepharo-conjunctivitis.

Sclera

The sclera is the white, fibrous, protective outer coating of the eye that is continuous with the cornea. The episclera is a thin layer of vascularized tissue that covers the sclera.

Episcleritis is a localized, elevated, and tender, but not usually painful, inflammation of the episclera (Fig. 6.62). It lasts for weeks and may be suppressed with topical steroid if itchy or uncomfortable. It is often a nonspecific immune response to surface irritants, but, infrequently, occurs in gout, syphilis, rheumatoid arthritis, and gastrointestinal disorders.

Scleritis is a severe inflammation of the sclera that may cause blindness. Unlike episcleritis, it is often painful. A quarter of the cases are associated with systemic immune or infectiois diseases such as systemic lupus erythematosis, rheumatoid arthritis, Lyme disease,

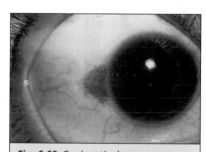

Fig. 6.60 Conjunctival nevus.

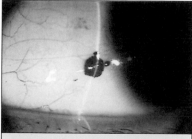

Fig. 6.61 Conjunctival melanoma.

tuberculosis, and syphilis, to name a few. Anterior scleritis is associated with visible engorgement of vessels deep to the conjunctiva (Fig. 6.63). Posterior scleritis causes choroidal effusions and even retinal detachments. Systemic corticosteroids, antimetabolites, or anti-infective drugs are usually required.

A blue sclera is due to increased scleral transparency, which allows choroidal pigment to be seen. It occurs normally in newborns, and abnormally in osteogenesis imperfecta (blue sclera with brittle bones), or following scleritis in rheumatoid arthritis (Fig. 6.64).

A staphyloma is a localized prolapse of bluish uveal tissue into thinned sclera. It occurs in rheumatoid arthritis, high myopia, or trauma (Fig. 6.65a).

Jaundice or icterus refers to yellowing of the skin or sclera due to increased levels of bilirubin (Fig. 6.65b). Because the elastin in the sclera has an increased affinity for bilirubin, it is often the first symptom of the condition. Total bilirubin is usually 0.3–1.0 mg/dl in adults and 1.0–12 mg/dl in newborns. Icterus first becomes toxic in adults above 12 mg/dl. Above this level, newborns could develop mental retardation; a condition called kernicterus.

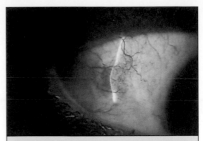

Fig. 6.62 Episcleritis. There is a 60% rate of recurrence.

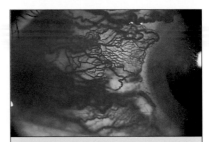

Fig. 6.63 Scleritis.

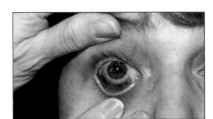

Fig. 6.64 Rheumatoid arthritis with thin sclera.

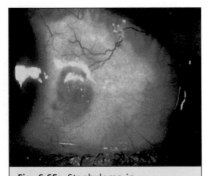

Fig. 6.65a Staphyloma in rheumatoid arthritis.

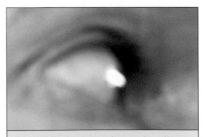

Fig. 6.65b Jaundice (icterus): yellow skin and sclera due to elevated bilirubin

Glaucoma

Glaucoma is a disease of the optic nerve most likely due to a compromised blood supply. The nerve can be damaged even more by elevated intraocular pressure pushing on the blood vessels supplying the nerve and causing a further reduction in blood flow.

Intraocular pressure is maintained by a balance between aqueous inflow and outflow. The aqueous produced by the ciliary body passes from the posterior chamber (the space behind the iris) through the pupil into the anterior chamber (Fig. 6.66). It drains through the trabecular meshwork and out of the eye through the venous canal of Schlemm (Figs 6.67a, b).

Glaucoma vs. glaucoma suspect

Normal intraocular pressure is 10–20 mmHg and should be measured at different times of day as there is a diurnal rhythm. Pressure greater than 28 mmHg should be treated to prevent loss of vision. Treat pressures of 20–27 mmHg when there is loss of vision, damage to the optic nerve, or a family history of glaucoma. Patients with pressures of 20–27 mmHg without these findings are called glaucoma suspects and are followed, but not treated.

Infrequently, the optic nerve could be damaged even when the pressure is less than 20 mmHg (normal tension glaucoma) and must be further reduced to the low teens.

Several instruments can be used to indirectly measure intraocular pressure by indenting the cornea.

A Goldmann applanation tonometer (Fig. 6.68) is the most accurate. It is used in conjunction with a slit lamp, and requires the use of anesthetic drops and fluorescein dye.

A Schiötz tonometer is a portable instrument (Fig. 6.69) that indents the anesthetized cornea and is used for bedside measurements.

The air-puff tonometer tests the pressure by blowing a puff of air at the eye. It is used by

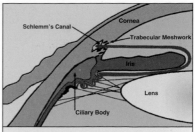

Fig. 6.66 Aqueous flow from ciliary body to Schlemm's canal. Courtesy of Pfizer Pharmaceuticals.

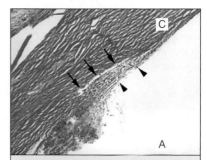

Fig. 6.67a Histology showing Schlemm's canal (↓↓), trabecular meshwork (↑↑), aqueous (A), and cornea (C).

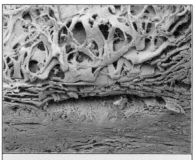

Fig. 6.67b Microscopic view of trabecular meshwork.

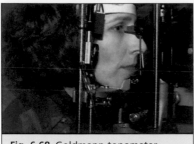

Fig. 6.68 Goldmann tonometer.

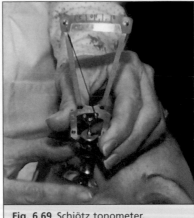

Fig. 6.69 Schiötz tonometer.

technicians since it does not require eye drops or corneal contact.

With all three instruments, the tonometric pressure reading is only an estimate of the real pressure. A thick cornea requires extra force to indent and, therefore, gives a falsely elevated reading, and the opposite is true with thin corneas. To better approximate the real pressure—especially in glaucoma suspects where exactitude is important—an ultrasonic pachymeter is used to measure corneal thickness. A conversion factor for corneal thickness then adjusts the tonometric reading upward or downward (Fig. 6.70).

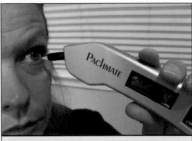

Fig. 6.70 Measurement of corneal thickness with ultrasonic pachymeter

The iridocorneal angle

Aqueous exits from the eye through the trabecular meshwork (Fig. 6.71) which is the tan to dark brown band at the angle between the cornea and iris. The angle, normally 15–45%, can be estimated with a slit lamp (Figs 6.72 and 6.73) but a goniolens (Figs 6.74 and 6.75) is more accurate. In open-angle glaucoma, the trabecular meshwork and the canal of Schlemm are obstructed, whereas in narrow-angle glaucoma, the space between the iris and cornea is too narrow so that aqueous cannot reach the trabecular meshwork. A narrow angle at risk of closing is graded 0–2. Angles of 3–4 are considered wide open with no chance of closing (Fig. 6.76).

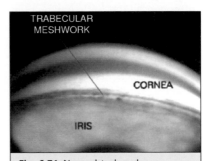

Fig. 6.71 Normal trabecular meshwork: grade 4 angle as seen with a goniolens.

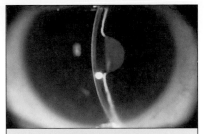

Fig. 6.72 Narrow angle in short hyperopic eye.

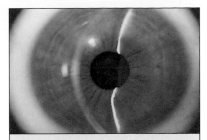

Fig. 6.73 Deep anterior chamber with wide open angle in long myopic eye.

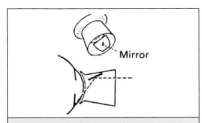

Mirror

Fig. 6.74 Trabecular meshwork seen with goniolens.

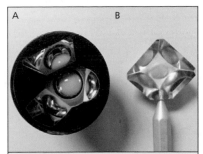

Fig. 6.75 A. Goldmann and B. Zeiss gonioscopic lenses used to examine the angle of the eye at the slit lamp.

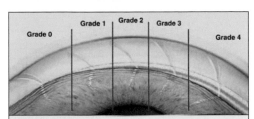

Grade 0 Grade 1 Grade 2 Grade 3 Grade 4

Fig. 6.76 Grading angle by progressive widening from 0–4. Courtesy of Pfizer Pharmaceuticals.

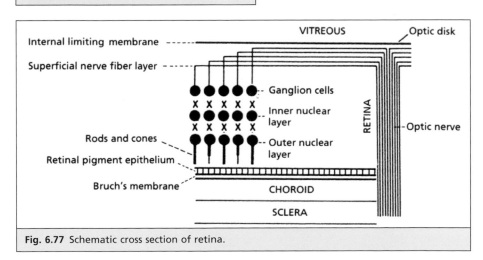

VITREOUS
Optic disk
Internal limiting membrane
Superficial nerve fiber layer
Ganglion cells
Inner nuclear layer
RETINA
Optic nerve
Rods and cones
Outer nuclear layer
Retinal pigment epithelium
Bruch's membrane
CHOROID
SCLERA

Fig. 6.77 Schematic cross section of retina.

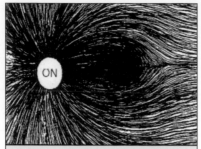

Fig. 6.78 Drawing of retinal nerve fiber layer with 1.2 million ganglion cell axons converging to make up the optic nerve (ON).

The optic disk (optic papilla)

The disk is the circular junction where the ganglion cell axons exit the eye, pick up a myelin sheath, and become the optic nerve (Figs 6.78 and 6.79). In the center of the optic disk is a cup that is usually less than one-third the disk diameter, although larger cups can be normal. As the pressure damages the nerve (Fig. 6.80):

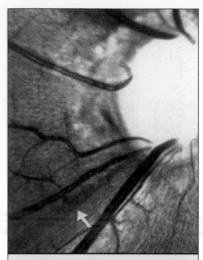

Fig. 6.79 "Red-free" photograph of glaucomatous cupping and loss of retinal nerve fiber layer (white arrows). The dark area with loss of striations is pathognomonic of fiber loss if it fans out and widens further from disk. Courtesy of Michael P. Kelly.

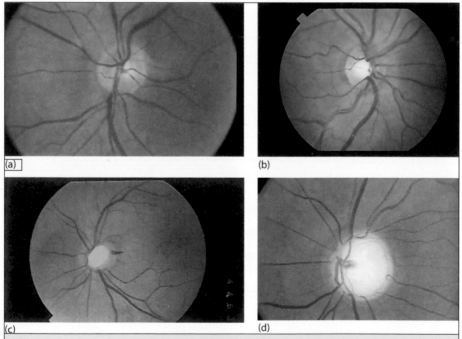

Fig. 6.80 Optic cup/disk ratio. (a) C/D = 0.25; (b) C/D = 0.40; (c) C/D = 0.70 with hemorrhage; (d) C/D = 0.90.

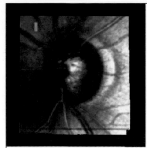
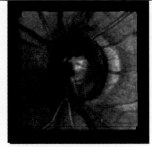
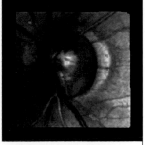

| Follow-Up: #3, Nov/30/1995 | Follow-Up: #6, May/9/1997 | Follow-Up: #9, Nov/24/1998 |

Fig. 6.81 Scanning laser optic disc topography with red color indicating progressive cupping over 3 year period. Courtesy of Heidelberg Engineering, Inc.

1 cup/disk ratio increases;

2 cup becomes more excavated and often unequal in the two eyes;

3 vessels shift nasally;

4 disk margin loses capillaries, turns pale, with infrequent flame hemorrhage (Fig. 6.80);

5 diffuse loss of retinal nerve fiber layer (Figs 6.81 and 6.82).

The optic disk changes can be followed by accurate drawings or photographs. Recently introduced, laser scanning tomography is more expensive but more accurately measures the three-dimensional changes in the optic disk (Fig. 6.80). Scanning laser polarimetry measures changes in the thickness of the nerve fiber layer around the disk (Fig. 6.81).

The latter test may be most useful for initial diagnosis. It is argued that if you wait for field defects before starting treatment, half the nerve fiber layer may already have been lost.

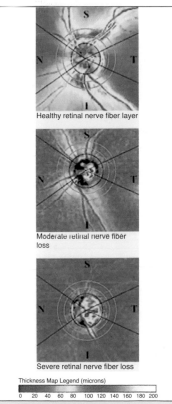

Healthy retinal nerve fiber layer

Moderate retinal nerve fiber loss

Severe retinal nerve fiber loss

Thickness Map Legend (microns)

0 20 40 60 80 100 120 140 160 180 200

Fig. 6.82 Color-coded GDx scanning laser polarimetry showing loss of thicker (yellow) nerve fiber layer over several years. It should be noted that the nerve fiber layer is normally thickest inferiorly then superiorly, followed by nasal, and then temporal. This can be remembered by the acronym ISN'T. Courtesy of Carl Zeiss Meditec, Inc.

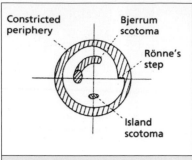

Fig. 6.83 Visual field defects in glaucoma.

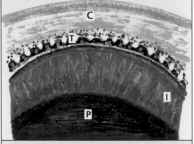

Fig. 6.84 Drawing of Argon laser trabeculoplasty. Up to 100 burns (white discoloration) may be applied to the junction of the pigmented and non-pigmented trabecular meshwork around the entire 360° circumference. The pressure lowering effect is likely due to the contraction of tissue around the trabecular meshwork stretching open the drainage pores. C, cornea; T, trabecular meshwork; I, iris; P, pupil.

Visual field defects pathognomonic of glaucoma

(Fig. 6.83)

1 Bjerrum's scotoma extends nasally from the blind spot in an arc.
2 Island defects could enlarge into a Bjerrum's scotoma.
3 Constricted fields occur before loss of central vision.
4 Ronne's nasal step is loss of peripheral nasal field above or below horizontal.

Therapy for open-angle glaucoma

The goal is to lower pressure below 20 mmHg, or at least to a level where there is no further loss of visual field or increase in cupping. Each patient should have a target pressure we try to attain and it is lowest in severe glaucoma. If optic nerve damage continues to progress even when pressures are maintained in the high teens, it is referred to as normal-tension glaucoma. The pressure in these eyes must be further decreased to the low teens. It may require a combination of medications, one from each of the classes on p. 94 or the addition of a surgical procedure (Figs 6.84–6.95).

Unfortunately, up to 60% of patients are noncomplaint in using their drops on schedule when using more than one drop.

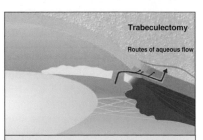

Fig. 6.85a Surgical trabeculectomy showing aqueous flow from cilliary body through iridectomy and scleral tunnel. It exits eye under conjunctiva. Courtesy of Pfizer Pharmaceuticals.

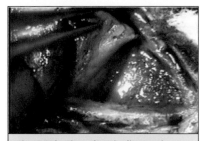

Fig. 6.85b The sclera is dissected toward the limbus to expose Schlemm's canal. Courtesy of iScience.

Surgical procedures for open-angle glaucoma

If maximum medical therapy does not control the pressure, surgery can be performed to increase aqueous outflow or less often to reduce aqueous secretion. Argon laser trabeculoplasty, which increases outflow, is often a first choice (Fig. 6.84). If pressure is still too high, a surgical hole is created at the limbus (trabeculectomy) to drain aqueous through the sclera and under the conjunctiva (Figs 6.85a–6.87).). The trabeculectomy could be repeated if the hole closes. If still unsuccessful, a tube could be implanted connecting the anterior chamber and subconjunctival space (Fig. 6.88). These two methods expose the interior of the eye of infection since only the conjunctiva protects it (Fig. 6.87).

Two new glaucoma surgeries have recently been introduced to increase aqueous outflow. The advantage of them is that unlike trabeculectomy, there is less risk of infection since they do not depend on a thin conjunctival flap. Neither of these two techniques has yet replaced trabeculectomy as the first line intraocular glaucoma surgery. Longer term follow-up is needed.

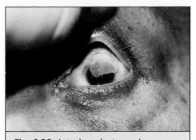

Fig. 6.86 A trabeculectomy is a surgically created fistula from anterior chamber to subconjunctival space. This bleb was too large and irritated the cornea and needs to be revised. Courtesy of Steven Brown, M.D. and *Arch. Ophth.*, Nov. 1999, Vol. 1, p. 1566, Copyright 1999, Amer. Med. Assoc.

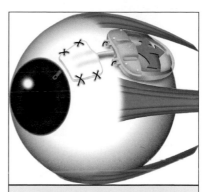

Fig. 6.88 Ahmed glaucoma valve. Tube in anterior chamber drains aqueous to subconjunctional space. Courtesy of New World Medical, Inc.

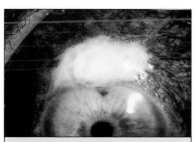

Fig. 6.87 The rate of trabeculectomy bleb-related infection is about 1.5% after two years, but is reported up to 8% when followed for longer periods. This conjunctival bleb was too thin and, got infected. The interior of this eye is at risk of endophthalmitis which could cause blindness. Courtesy of Donald L. Bendenz and *Arch. Ophth.* Aug. 1999, Vol. 117, p. 1010, Copyright 1999, Amer. Med. Assoc.

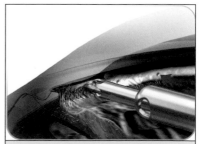

Fig. 6.89 Trabectome unroofing Schlemm's canal. Invented by Roy Chuck, MD and George Baerveldt, MD. Albert Einstein Medical School.

Common glaucoma medications and side effects

Class and action	Chemical name	Trade name	Generic Available (G) Concentration	Dosage	Comment
Beta-blocker ↓Aqueous secretion	Betaxolol (G)	Betopic S	0.25%	BID	Slows heart rate Aggravates respiratory conditions
	Timolol (G) Timoptic gel (G)	Timoptic, Betimol Timoptic-XE	0.25% & 0.50% 0.25% & 0.50%	BID QD	Betoptic is cardioselective with least systemic side effects
Prostaglandin analogue ↑Aqueous outflow	Latanoprost (G) Travoprost Bimatoprost	Xalatan Travatan Z Lumigan	0.005% 0.004% 0.01%	HS	Darkening and lengthening of eyelashes, with hyperpigmentation of iris and periocular (eyelid) skin (Figs 11–12). Also iritis, macular edema, and conjunctivitis
Alpha adrenergic agonist ↓Aqueous secretion ↑Aqueous outflow	Brimonidine (G) 0.15 and 0.2%	Alphagan P	0.1% 0.15%	TID	Frequent allergy
Carbonic anhydrase inhibitor Topical	Dorzolamide (G)	Trusopt	2% ophth sol	TID	Could suppress bone marrow
	Brinzolamide	Azopt	1% ophth sol	TID	
Oral ↓Aqueous secretion	Acetazolamide (G)	Diamox	250 mg 500 mg tablet	250 mg (QID) 500 mg (BID)	Could suppress bone marrow
Cholinergic ↑Aqueous outflow	Pilocarpine (G)	Pilocar	0.5–6.0%	QID	Retinal detachment, cataracts, small pupil, brow ache
Combination*	Timolol and Dorzolamide (G)	Cosopt	0.5 and 2%	BID	
	Brimonidine 0.2% Timolol 0.5%	Combigan	0.2 and 0.5%		Convenient

* Xalatan, Lumigan, or Travatan, combined with Timolol awaiting approval in USA.

One technique uses an electrosurgical-pulsed instrument called trabectome. It vaporizes about 90° of diseased trabecular tissue that is obstructing access to Schlemm's canal (Figs 6.89–6.91).

The other new procedure is called canaloplasty (Figs 6.92 and 6.93). In this technique a suture is placed in Schlemm's canal and then tied and tightened to stretch it open.

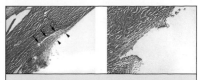

Fig. 6.90 Schlemm's canal (↓↓↓), Trabecular meshwork (↑↑).

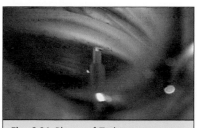

Fig. 6.91 Photo of Trabectome.

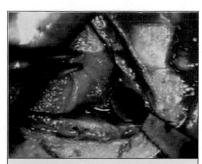

Fig. 6.92 Dissection of sclera to wards the limbus. A window of the sclera is then removed for entry into Schlemm's canal.

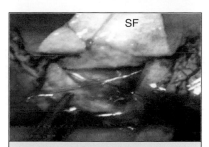

Fig. 6.93a Canaloplasty: A scleral flap (SF) is created to expose Schlemm's canal. A microcatheter then threaded into Schlemm's canal. It is then withdrawn dragging a suture with it that remains in place.

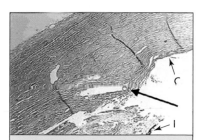

Fig. 6.93b Histology of the angle between the cornea (C), and the iris (I) showing suture in Schlemm's canal.

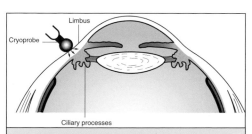

Fig. 6.94 Transscleral cryotherapy is applied for less than 20 seconds to 180° of sclera 1mm posterior to limbus.

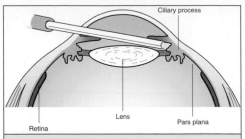

Fig. 6.95 Endoscopic cyclophotocoagulation for partial destruction of aqueous secreting ciliary processes. One probe consisting of a light source, laser, and camera is usually inserted into the eye near the corneal limbus although a pars plana site may be used. Anywhere from 170–280° is usually treated.

The previously discussed surgeries increased aqueous outflow from the eye.

Another strategy is to surgically reduce aqueous production by destroying some of the ciliary processes. To accomplish this, transscleral "cryo" or laser therapy may be applied to the area directly overlying the ciliary processes (Fig. 6.94).

A newer technique called endoscopic cyclophotocoagulation is performed by entering the eye and destroying the ciliary process with direct visualization (Fig. 6.95)

Angle-closure glaucoma

Angle-closure glaucoma is less common than the previously discussed open-angle glaucoma and its treatment is different. It usually occurs in hyperopic eyes that are short with crowded anterior segments. The iris in these eyes is closer to the cornea (see Fig. 6.72). The resulting narrow angle becomes even more narrow when the pupil becomes mid-dilated. In this position, there is maximum contact between the iris and lens preventing the aqueous from reaching the anterior chamber and the trabecular meshwork. This "pupillary block" traps aqueous behind the iris and pushes the iris forward even more until the angle is totally closed.

The total closure of the angle causes a sudden elevation in pressure, often exceeding 60 mmHg. This pressure damages the pupil, causing it to remain fixed and dilated.

Symptoms include pain, blurred vision, halos, and nausea. Signs include a mid-dilated non-reactive pupil, corneal edema, and a reddened conjunctiva (Figs 6.96 and 6.97).

The pupil dilation precipitating this attack may be caused by stimulation of the pupillary dilator muscle by adrenergic drugs, stress, or darkness. Anti-cholinergic drugs, such as major tranquilizers, block the sphincter muscle and may trigger an attack.

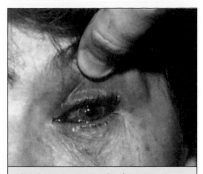

Fig. 6.96 Acute angle-closure glaucoma with dilated pupil.

Treatment of angle-closure glaucoma first requires lowering of the pressure to break the attack and clear the cornea. It usually includes pilocarpine 1% to constrict the pupil and up to three other pressure lowering drops. If the pressure still remains too high, a short acting hyperosmotic agent such as mannitol 20% i.v. or oral glycerine 50% may be administered. Both draw fluid out of the eye by increasing the osmolarity of the blood. Once the attack is arrested, the corneal edema clears so that a laser iridotomy can be performed (Fig. 6.98). This allows aqueous to

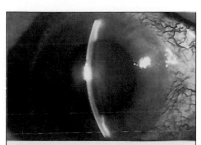

Fig. 6.97 Angle-closure glaucoma: shallow anterior chamber and corneal edema.

Common types of glaucoma

	Primary open-angle	Angle-closure
Occurrence	70% of all glaucomas	10% of all glaucomas
Etiology	Unknown obstruction in trabecular meshwork, usually inherited; increases with age	Closed angle increases with age and hyperopia
Symptoms	Usually asymptomatic	Red, painful eye; halos around lights; nausea
Signs	Elevated pressure Increased disk cupping Visual field defect	Markedly elevated pressure Steamy cornea Fixed, mid-dilated pupil Conjunctival injection
Treatment	Usually eye drops	Laser iridotomy
Contraindicated medications	Corticosteroids—high doses or long-term use mandate pressure testing	Pupil dilators such as adrenergics, anticholinergics, antihistamines, major tranquilizers

flow into the anterior chamber and bypass the pupillary block. It is often a permanent cure and the pupil may then be safely dilated.

Less common types of glaucoma, called secondary open-angle glaucoma, could be caused by blockage of the trabecular meshwork by pigment (Fig. 6.99), hemorrhage, inflammatory cells (as in iritis), pseudoexfoliation (Fig. 6.100), or scarring from rubeosis iridis (Figs 6.119 and 6.120).

Trauma could cause glaucoma by tearing the iris at its insertion on the ciliary body. Often, there is associated bleeding in the anterior chamber (Fig. 6.101) referred to as a hyphema. Complications of hyphema include rebleeds, associated retinal damage, and glaucoma. Rx: bilateral patch and absolute bedrest for 5 days.

Gonioscopy may reveal angle recession (Fig. 6.102) in which the iris insertion is torn posteriorly, exposing a wide band of darkly pigmented ciliary body. Patients should be monitored indefinitely since about 10% ultimately develop glaucoma.

Congenital glaucoma is fortunately rare, but must be suspected since routine office eye pressure measurements are difficult, if not impossible, in infants and young children. Clues to arouse suspicion are squinting, tearing, an enlarged globe (buphthalmos) (Fig. 6.104), and corneal edema. The latter may cause a subtle loss of a normally shiny, clear corneal surface (Fig. 6.103). It is due to

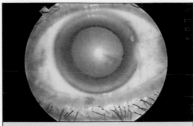

Fig. 6.98 Peripheral iridotomy at 2 o'clock.

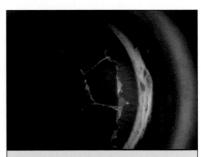

Fig. 6.100 Pseudoexfoliation is identified by white flakes on the anterior lens capsule, pupillary margin, zonules, and trabecular meshwork. It is relatively common and is associated with an increased incidence of glaucoma and weakened zonules which could complicate cataract surgery.
Courtesy of Rhonda Curtis, CRA, COT Washington Univ. Medical School St. Louis, Missouri and J. Ophthal. Photography

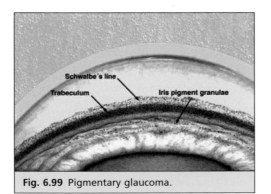

Schwalbe's line

Trabeculum

Iris pigment granulae

Fig. 6.99 Pigmentary glaucoma.

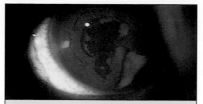

Fig. 6.101 Hyphema with large iris disinsertion (dialysis) from its root.

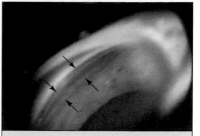

Fig. 6.102 Angle recessed posteriorly following traumatic hyphema. The recessed angle is seen as a wide dark band between the cornea and the iris (↑).

the damaging effect of the pressure on the corneal endothelium.

One type of juvenile glaucoma occurs in Sturge-Weber syndrome (Fig. 4.46) in which there are angiomatosis of the face and meninges with cerebral calcifications and seizures.

Uvea (Figs 6.105 and 6.106)

The uvea is composed of the iris, ciliary body and choroid. All three are contiguous, and pigmented with melanocytes.

The iris is a diaphragm that changes the size of the pupil by the action of the sympatheic dilator m. and the cholinergic constrictor m.

The ciliary body (Figs 6.106–6.108) is made up of the four clinically significant parts.

1. The anterior region serves as the site for insertion of the iris.

2. The ciliary processes secrete the aqueous.

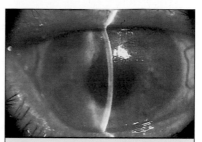

Fig. 6.103 Glaucoma causing a cloudy, edematous cornea.

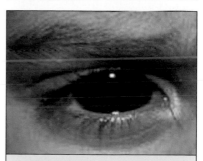

Fig. 6.104 Congenital glaucoma in an 8 month old causing squinting, an enlarged globe, and subtle corneal edema causing an obscured view of the iris. Courtesy of Karen Joos, MD, PhD, Vanderbilt Eye Instit., Nashville, TN.

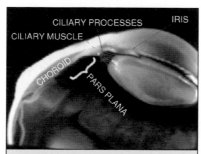

CILIARY PROCESSES   IRIS
CILIARY MUSCLE
CHOROID PARS PLANA

Fig. 6.105 Uvea. Courtesy of Stephen McCormick.

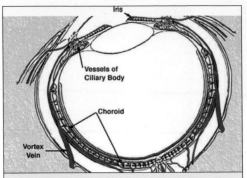

Fig. 6.106 The uvea is made up of the iris, ciliary body, and choroid. Courtesy of Pfizer Pharmaceuticals.

3. The smooth muscle changes the focus of the lens by contracting and decreasing tension on the zonules (Fig. 6.108).

4. The avascular and flat pars plana serves as the best location to surgically enter the eye for vitreoretinal surgery (Fig. 7.90 and 7.91).

The choroid is highly vascularized and nourishes retinal rods, cones, and pigment epithelium. Unlike the tree-like branching of the retinal vessels, the choroidal circulation appears to be criss-crossing in a tigroid-like appearance (Fig. 6.109). It is most easily visualized in advanced dry macular degeneration after the retinal pigment layer disappears (Fig. 7.46) or in albinism where the retinal pigment never fully developed (Fig. 7.62).

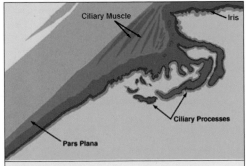

Fig. 6.107 Ciliary body. Courtesy of Pfizer Pharmaceuticals.

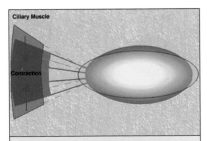

Fig. 6.108 Ciliary muscle focusing lens. Courtesy of Pfizer Pharmaceuticals.

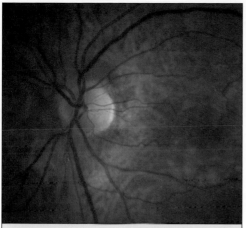

Fig. 6.109 Tigroid fundus with clearly visible choroidal vasculature. Courtesy of Elliot Davidoff, M.D.

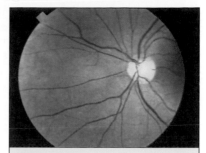

Fig. 6.110 Flat benign choroidal nevus.

Malignant melanoma

A melanocyte tumor is the most common primary intraocular malignancy. It is unilateral and develops from the choroid in 85% of cases, the ciliary body in 9%, and the iris in 6%. Choroidal lesions are elevated and usually slate gray, but may be white to black with yellow–gold and uneven pigmentation (Fig. 6.111) unlike a benign nevus, which is usually a more uniform gray color and flat (Fig. 6.110). This must be distinguished from metastatic carcinoma to the eye, which is also most common in the choroid but is usually lighter in color. The primary site is most often the breast or lung. Small intraocular malignancies are usually treated with a radioactive plaque (Fig. 6.112) which may preserve some vision. For larger tumors, the eye is sometimes removed (Figs 6.113, 6.114 and 6.151). If the tumor extends beyond the globe and is life threatening, an exenteration of the orbit is required. This rarely performed surgery is disfiguring and destructive. It could necessitate removal of the orbital contents, the eyelids, orbital walls, and periorbital structures (Fig. 6.115).

Patients with melanoma of the skin and elsewhere are often referred to eye physicians to rule out the eye as a primary site or a site of metastasis.

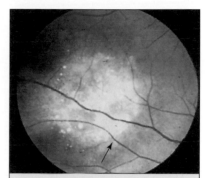

Fig. 6.111 Elevated malignant choroidal melanoma. Note change in direction as artery rises over tumor (↑).

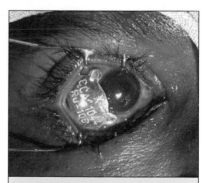

Fig. 6.112 Radioactive plaque sewn or glued to the episclera of the eye is usually left in place for about 4 days and is used to treat smaller intraocular tumors. Courtesy of Dr. Santosh G. Honor and Dr. Surbhi Joshi, Prasad Eye Institute, Hyderabad, India.

Benign iris freckles (Fig. 6.116) and nevi are common, whereas malignant iris melanoma (Figs 6.117 and 6.118) is extremely rare. Lesions become more suspicious if they are growing, elevated, vascularized, distort the pupil, or cause inflammation, glaucoma, or cataracts.

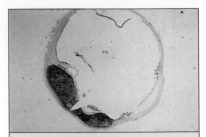

Fig. 6.113 Gross section of malignant melanoma treated with removal of eye (enucleation).

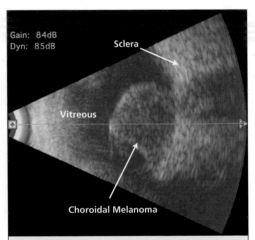

Fig. 6.114 B-scan ultrasound of a malignant choroidal melanoma showing typical dome-shaped growth which helps to confirm the diagnosis. The scan also shows its size and whether it extends beyond the sclera which will determine the type of treatment. This eye, with this massive tumor, was enucleated.

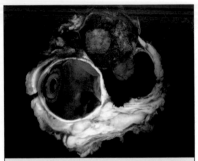

Fig. 6.115 Exenteration of the orbit for malignant melanoma extending beyond the sclera. Reproduced from *Brit. J. Ophthal.* Vol. 94, Issue 5, May 2010, Massive orbital recurrence or uveal melanoma without metastases after 28 years. Jonathan J. Ross, Simon J. Dean, David A. Koppel, Fiona Roberts, Ewan G. Kemp with permission from BMJ Publishing Group, Ltd.

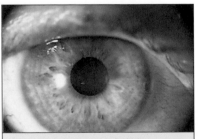

Fig. 6.116 Benign iris freckle.

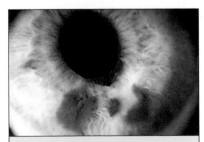

Fig. 6.117 Malignant iris melanoma with elevated lesions and distorted pupil.

Rubeosis iridis is a serious condition in which abnormal vessels grow on the surface of the iris (Figs 6.119 and 6.120) in response to ischemia associated with central retinal vein occlusion, proliferative diabetic retinopathy, or carotid artery occlusive disease. Laser photocoagulation of the retina may cause regression of iris vessels. Untreated, the neovascularization could cause severe glaucoma.

An iris coloboma (Fig. 6.121) is due to failure of embryonic tissue to fuse inferiorly. It may also involve the choroid, lens, and optic nerve.

Inflammations of the uvea are categorized by location. A. anterior (iritis), B. intermediate (ciliary body-cyclitis), C. posterior (chorioretinitis), and D. panuveitis involving all uveal structures. In 50% of cases, no cause is found. Most are treated with steriods and, less often, with non-steroidal anti-inflammatories (NSAID). An immunomodulator, most often, methotrexate is sometimes required.

A. Iritis, inflammation of the iris, accounts for 92% of cases of uveitis. It causes pain, tearing, and photophobia. Signs include miosis (small pupil), perilimbal conjunctival injection (Figs 6.122 and 6.125), and anterior chamber flare and cells (Fig. 6.123). Flare refers to the beam's milky appearance due to elevated protein. With the slit lamp on high magnification and a short, bright beam shone across the dark pupil, inflammatory cells are graded from trace to very many (4+).

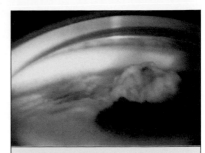

Fig. 6.118 Gonioscopic view of elevated iris melanoma. Courtesy of Michael P. Kelly.

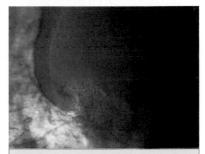

Fig. 6.119 Rubeosis iridis.

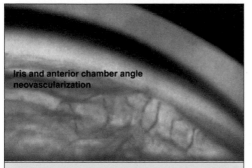

Iris and anterior chamber angle neovascularization

Fig. 6.120 Rubeosis iridis. These abnormal iris blood vessels scar the angle of the eye. They most often result from ischemic retinal diseases such as proliferative diabetic retinopathy and central retinal artery or vein occlusion.

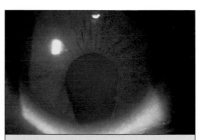

Fig. 6.121 Iris coloboma.

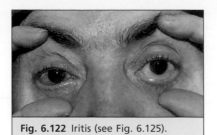

Fig. 6.122 Iritis (see Fig. 6.125).

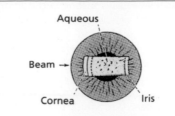

Fig. 6.123 Slit-beam view of flare and cells in anterior chamber.

Deposits of inflammatory cells and protein on the corneal endothelium (Figs 6.124, 6.125 and 6.128) are called keratitic precipitates (KPs) and are often a sign of chronicity. Iritis usually reduces eye pressure due to depressed secretion of aqueous and increased uveoscleral outflow. Eye pressure may become elevated if cellular debris obstructs the trabecular meshwork, or from the steroid used to treat the uveitis.

Another complication of iritis is posterior synechiae. These are adhesions between the iris and the lens capsule (Fig. 6.124a). To prevent this, drops are used to keep the pupil dilated and steroids are given to prevent a fibrinous sticky aqueous.

Treatment for iritis includes a topical cycloplegic such as cyclogel 1% and a steroid such as Pred Forte 1%. Frequency and strength of medication depends on the severity of the condition. Besides dilating the pupil, the cycloplegic also relieves the pain due to ciliary muscle spasm spasm.

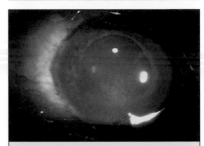

Fig. 6.124a Keratitic precipitates and posterior synechiae.

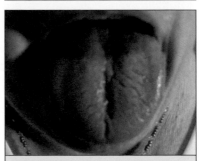

Fig. 6.124b Patient with Behcet's disease with ulcers and fissures on her tongue. She complained of constant burning in mouth.

Anticholinergic	Action time	Primary use
Atropine 0.5–1%	±2 weeks	Prolonged or severe anterior uveitis
Scopolamine 0.25% (hyoscine 0.25%)	±4 days	Alternative when allergic to atropine
Homatropine 2–5%	±2 days	Anterior uveitis
Cyclopentolate (Cyclogel) 1–2%	±1 day	Cycloplegic retinoscopy; rapid onset (30 min)
Tropicamide (Mydriacyl) 0.5%	±6 hours	Often used with phenylephrine 2.5% or 10% for pupil dilation.

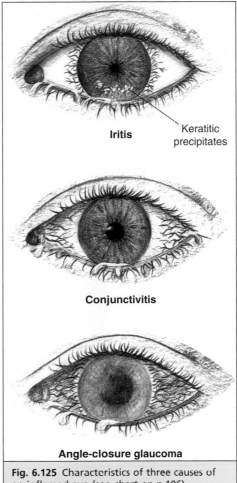

Iritis

Keratitic precipitates

Conjunctivitis

Angle-closure glaucoma

Fig. 6.125 Characteristics of three causes of an inflamed eye (see chart on p.106).

Iritis is caused most often by intraocular surgery, blunt ocular trauma, and corneal ulcers, abrasions, and foreign bodies. Human leukocyte antigen (HLA-B27) is found in 2–9% of normal persons. In this small group of individuals possessing the HLA-B27 antigen, 20% are predisposed to autoimmune disorders. Iritis may be associated with the following five HLA-B27 positive autoimmune diseases:

1. Ankylosing spondylitis (males with arthritis of the lower spine — 95% are HLA-B27 positive)
2. Juvenile idiopathic arthritis
3. Reactive arthritis (formerly Reiter's syndrome), in males with urethritis and conjunctivitis.

4. Inflammatory bowel disease
5. Psoriatic arthritis.

Causes that are not related to HLA-B27 levels are toxoplasmosis, sarcoidosis, Lyme disease, influenza, lymphoma, AIDS, herpes simplex and zoster (shingles), and Behcet's disease (ulcers in the mouth [Fig 6.124b] and genitals). There are other even rarer etiologies. Therefore, careful clinical judgement is needed in determining the timing and extent of the work-up, taking into consideration cost, severity, chronicity, and associated medical history. (See p. 114 and 115 for basic work-up)

Patients with juvenile idiopathic arthritis and chronic iritis often develop a band of calcification in Bowman's membrane known as band keratopathy (Fig. 6.126). It also occurs in sarcoidosis and hypervitaminosis D. It may be removed by using a technique called chelation in which the calcium is dissolved by applying diamine-tetra-acetic (EDTA) to the cornea.

B. Inflammation of the ciliary body (cyclitis), also called intermediate uveitis, is characterized 80% of the time by having cells in the vitreous. It causes pain and decreased eye pressure. Cells in the vitreous reduce vision. Multiple sclerosis, sarcoidosis (Figs 6.127 and 6.128) and cigarette smoking are the commonly associated causes.

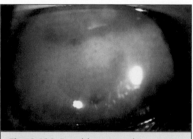

Fig. 6.126 Band keratopathy.

COMMON CAUSES OF AN INJECTED CONJUNCTIVA

	Iritis	Conjunctivitis	Acute glaucoma
Symptom	Pain, photophobia	Gritty, itching	Pain (often severe), photophobia
Discharge	Tearing	Pus, mucus, or tears	Tearing
Pupil	Miotic	Normal	Mid-dilated
Injection	Limbal	Diffuse	Diffuse & limbal
Cornea	Keratitic precipitates	Clear	Steamy cornea
Pressure	Usually low	Normal	Elevated
Anterior chamber	Flare and cells	Normal	Shallow

Anti-inflammatories

Aside from their use in uveitis, steroids are also commonly used to treat post-operative inflammation, conjunctivitis, keratitis, scleritis, episcleritis, macular edema, giant cell arteritis, and Grave's orbitopathy. They may be given orally, by eye drop, subconjunctival injection, and intravitreal implant or injection. Choose the route and lowest dosage to minimize side effects.

Local side effects of corticosteroids include cataracts, glaucoma, and activation of herpes keratitis. Systemic side effects include reduced immunity, osteoporosis, or exacerbation of diabetes or gastric ulcers. Topical non-steroidal anti-inflammatory drops (NSAIDs), such as generic ketorolac (Acular), are less effective and may be used an alternate treatment or added to steroid, especially in glaucoma patients since they don't elevate eye pressure.

Sarcoidosis

Sarcoidosis is a systemic disease of unknown etiology characterized in 75% of patients by granulomatous inflammation of the lung (Fig. 6.127). It also affects skin (Fig. 6.128), peripheral nerves, liver, kidney, and other tissues. The main ocular finding is iritis often associated with large, greasy (mutton-fat) keratitic precipitates (Fig. 6.128). Lacrimal gland granulomas (Figs 6.131 and 6.132), intermediate uveitis (Figs 6.129 and 6.130) vasculitis and (Fig. 6.135) occur less frequently. It is usually treated with local or systemic corticosteroids.

C. Choroiditis is characterized by white exudates extending onto the retina, sometimes obscured from view by cells in the vitreous. It leads to chorioretinal atrophy with pigment mottling (Fig. 6.133). Often no cause is found, but the following etiologies should be considered:

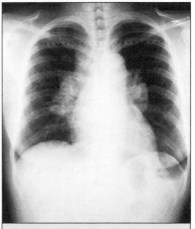

Fig. 6.127 Hilar adenopathy is the number one sign of sarcoidosis occuring in 75% of cases. Courtesy of Aman K. Farr, M.D. and *Arch. Ophth.*, May 2000, Vol. 118, No. 1–6 p. 729. Copyright 2000, Amer. Med. Assoc. All rights reserved.

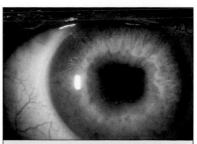

Fig. 6.128 Iritis occurs in 25% of patients with sarcoidosis and is the number one ocular finding. Above are large smooth (mutton-fat) keratitic precipitates and an irregular pupil due to posterior synechiae. Courtesy of Rhonda Curtis, CRA, COT, Washington Univ. Medical School, St. Louis MO.

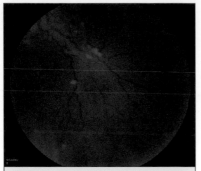

Fig. 6.129 Sarcoidosis with intermediate uveitis and "snowballs" of inflammatory cells in the peripheral vitreous. Courtesy of Julia Monsonego, CRA Wills Eye Hospital.

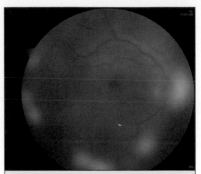

Fig. 6.130 Intermediate uveitis (pars planitis) with snowbanking of inflammatory cells on the pars plana. Courtesy of Careen lowder, MD, Cole Eye Institute.

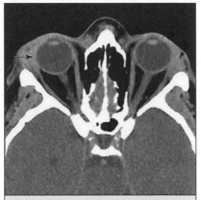

Fig. 6.131a CT scan of sarcoidosis with bilaterally enlarged lacrimal glands (↑). This patient also had lung, skin, conjunctiva, and kidney involvement.

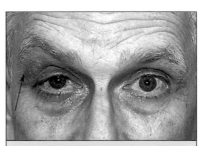

Fig. 6.131b Visibly enlarged right lacrimal gland (↑). Notice elevated right brow and ptosis.

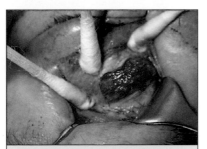

Fig. 6.132 A lacrimal gland biopsy often helps confirm the diagnosis of sarcoidosis.

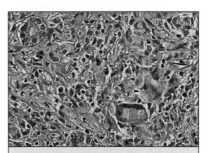

Fig. 6.133 Light photomicrograph of lacrimal gland infiltrated with noncaseating granuloma.

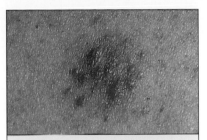

Fig. 6.134 Tender erythematous subcutaneous sarcoid nodule (Figs 6.131a-6.134). Courtesy of Dr. John Woogend and *Arch. Ophth.*, May 2007, Vol 125 p. 707–709.

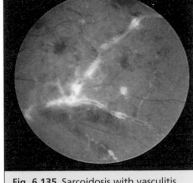

Fig. 6.135 Sarcoidosis with vasculitis causing "candle-wax" drippings on vessel. Courtesy of Joseph Walsh. M.D.

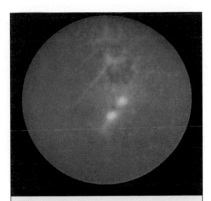

Fig. 6.136a Toxoplasma gondii choroidiosis often reactivates next to lesion. One quarter of the US population is seropositive for toxoplasmosis, but only 2% of these will develop eye disease. Up to 25% of lamb and pork in the US has been reported to harbor cysts. Infection is spread by congenital or oral transmission.

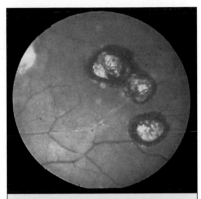

Fig. 6.136b Old toxoplasmosis scar: sclera visible through atrophic retina and choroid.

Causes of choroiditis

1 Bacterial: syphilis, (Fig. 6.139) tuberculosis
2 Viral: herpes simplex, cytomegalovirus in 25% of AIDS patients (Figs 6.147, 7.56)
3 Fungal: histoplasmosis (Fig. 6.137), candidiasis
4 Parasitic: Toxoplasma, Toxocara (Fig. 6.138)
5 Immunosuppresssion: AIDS predisposes to several of above
6 Autoimmune: Behcet's disease (mouth and genital ulcers with dermatitis); sympathetic ophthalmia.

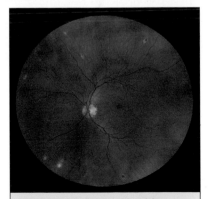

Fig. 6.137 Histoplasmosis with multiple punched out chorioretinitic lesions called "histo spots". Courtesy of Alexis Smith, CRT, OCT-T, Kellogg Eye Center, Michigan.

Choroiditis often requires subconjunctival, intravitreal, or systemic steroid, especially when it threatens the macula, optic nerve, or the associated vitritis is a potential source of membrane formation and decreased vision.

Nematodes

Parasitic worms, sometimes referred to as microfilaria, may infect humans. *Toxocara canis* and *cati* (Fig. 6.138) are microfilaria transmitted by the oral ingestion of ova. Toddlers may ingest them by playing on the ground where these animals defecated and adults by eating unwashed vegetables.

Don't confuse the toxocara nematode that is an extracellular parasite with the other similar sounding parasite, toxoplasmosis, which lives inside the cell. However, what toxocara and toxoplasmosis have in common is that both may cause severe intraocular inflammation resulting in blindness.

Onchocerca volvulus, found 95% of the time in Africa afflicts people living along riverbanks. It's responsible for 270,000 cases of blindness caused by scarring of the cornea, optic neuritis, and choroiditis. The disease is often called "river blindness". Another African worm – loa loa – can migrate to the lids and conjunctiva where they can live for up to 17 years and cause inflammation.

Syphilis (Figs 6.139–6.143)

This infectious disease caused by *Treponema pallidum* is usually transmitted through sexual contact. It can infect any organ of the body. Ocular involvement usually includes the uvea resulting in iritis, cyclitis, and chorioretinitis. Neurosyphilis could involve all the cranial nerves and cause the pupillary response called the Argyll Robertson pupil.

Here the pupils may be irregularly constricted with decreased or absent response to light, but a normal near reflex. The pupil dilates poorly with mydriatics.

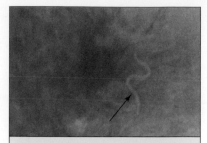

Fig. 6.138 Unknown southeastern U.S. subretinal nematode (↑) causing neuroretinitis. Courtesy of J. Donald M. Gass, MD and *Arch. Ophth.*, Nov. 1983, Vol. 101 3, p. 1689–1697.

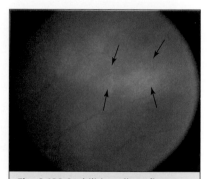

Fig. 6.139 Syphilitic, yellow, flat chorioretinal lesions. Courtesy of Thomas R. Friberg, M.D. and *Arch. Ophth.*, Nov. 1989, Vol. 107, p. 1571–1572.

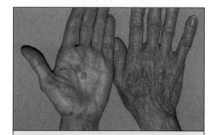

Fig. 6.140 Maculopapular syphilitic eruption involving palms.

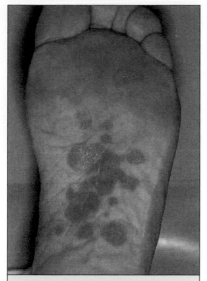

Fig. 6.141 Maculopapular syphilitic eruption involving soles.

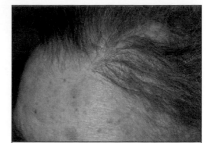

Fig. 6.142 Zones of alopecia prompted patient to wear a wig.

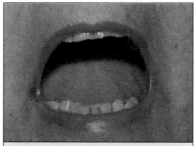

Fig. 6.143 Painless mucous membrane ulcers occurred at the corners of patient's mouth.

Sadly, in the last decade, the incidence of syphilis has increased in males having sex with males.

Human immunodeficiency virus (HIV)

This retrovirus invades and inactivates the CD4-T lymphocytes of the immune system. Initially, it may cause weight loss, headache, malaise, fever, chills, and lymphadenopathy. When the CD4-T cells drop from the normal of 500–1500 cells/mm to less than 200, the acquired immune deficiency syndrome (AIDS) begins. AIDS occurs in 38.3% of those infected with HIV within a year of diagnosis and 45% within three years. Up to 90% of adults in the US harbor herpes simplex virus; 40 to 80% have cytomegalovirus (CMV) (Fig. 6.147); and 25% have +antibodies to *Toxoplasmosis gondii*. These three organisms are among the

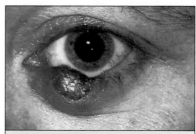

Fig. 6.144 Kaposi's sarcoma of skin in AIDS due to the opportunistic infection herpes virus 8. Courtesy of Jerry Shields, MD.

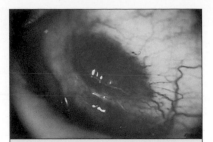

Fig. 6.145 Kaposi's sarcoma of conjunctiva. Courtesy of Jerry Shields, MD.

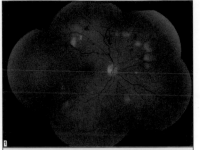

Fig. 6.146 AIDS retinopathy with cotton wool spots and intraretinal hemorrhages occurs in 50% of patients with AIDS. There is no treatment Courtesy of Julia Monsonego, CRA Wills Eye Hospital.

most common to become virulent in immuno-compromised patients with AIDS.

If the CD4+T count is >200 cells/mm with no ocular disease, a yearly eye exam is adequate. IF CD4+T is <50 cells/mm, the eye exam should be every 4 months. If on highly active antiretroviral therapy (HAART), the patient should be checked more often since the medications or the disease could cause uveitis, vitritis, epiretinal membranes, or acute retinal necrosis that could lead to retinal detachment. HAART therapy, together with Vitrasert (ganciclovir) intravitreal implants, have resulted in a reduction in both HIV and CMV associated mortality and a 90% reduction in retinitis complications in the US.

Kaposi's sarcoma (Figs 6.144 and 145) is a malignancy seen most often in AIDS. There is a non-tender purple nodule on the skin or conjunctiva. Rx: radiation or excision.

Sympathetic ophthalmia is a rare condition. It refers to a traumatic or surgical injury to the

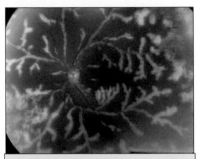

Fig. 6.147 Cytomegalovirus (CMV) is the most frequent opportunistic infection in patients with AIDs and the retinitis is a significant risk factor for mortality. This case shows frosted retinal angitis. Courtesy of Harry Flynn, MD and Retinal Physician, Oct. 2010, Vol. 7, No. 8, p. 67.

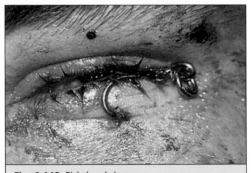

Fig. 6.148 Fish hook in eye.

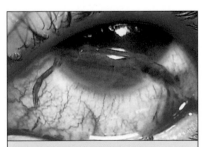

Fig. 6.149 Open globe injury through corneoscleral wall with prolapse of iris and ciliary body.

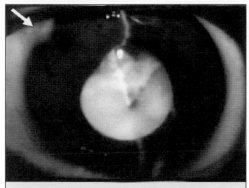

Fig. 6.150 Penetrating injury through iris and lens capsule with secondary cataract.

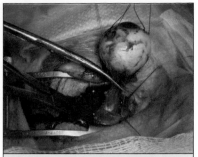

Fig. 6.151 Enucleation: The eye is removed by first exposing and then severing the insertions of the six extraocular mm. Then the optic n. is cut as shown above. An eye may be removed when it is blind, painful, cosmetically unappealing, or harbors a tumor. Courtesy of Jeffrey Nerad, MD

uvea of one eye causing an immune uveitis in the uninvolved eye. A penetrating injury through the corneoscleral wall is referred to as an open globe injury (Fig. 6.149). Handle the eye with minimal probing. Place the patient at rest with bilateral shields that exert no pressure; start IV broad spectrum antibiotics; and call the eye surgeon immediately. If the uvea or retina are extruded from the eye and it cannot be repaired, the eye is removed (enucleated) (Fig. 6.151). A spherical prosthesis is then placed in the orbit and covered with conjunctiva (Figs 6.152–6.154). A removable scleral prosthesis painted to match the other eye is placed on the conjunctiva. Enucleation should be performed within 10 days of the injury to prevent sympathetic ophthalmia.

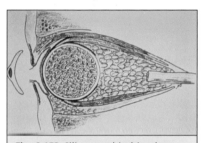

Fig. 6.152 Silicone orbital implant with scleral prosthesis. Courtesy of Integrated Orbital Implants, Inc.

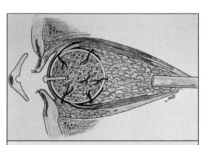

Fig. 6.153 Porous hydroxyapatite implant allows ingrowth of blood vessels to prevent migration or extrusion. Addition of the peg allows more normal movement, but has more complications. Courtesy of Integrated Orbital Implants, Inc.

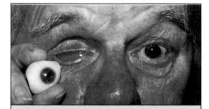

Fig. 6.154 Enucleated socket with scleral prosthesis.

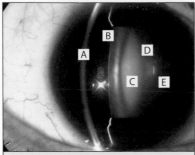

Fig. 6.155 Slit lamp view of lens: A-cornea, B-anterior capsule, C-nucleus, D-posterior cortex E-posterior capsule. Courtesy of Takashi Fujkado, MD

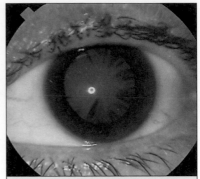

Fig. 6.156 Anterior cortical spokes.

A work-up for uveitis is necessary when there is no obvious cause and if it is prolonged or severe. The following screening tests for most common causes should be considered depending on the geographic location, age of patient, and other signs and symptoms. The patient should also be referred to a primary care physician suggesting reasons for this work-up with your recommendations.

Diagnosis	Major clues	Laboratory evaluation
AIDS	Malaise, weight loss, lymphadenopathy, and signs of infection, especially toxoplasmosis, cytomegalovirus, and herpes simplex	HIV-1, HIV-2, antibody screen
Ankylosing spondylitis	Often males with lower back pain	HLA-B27, sacroiliac and lumbar spinal x-ray
Anterior uveitis (HLA-B27+)	Associated with ankylosing spondylitis, inflammatory bowel disease, psoriasis, Reiter's syndrome, juvenile idiopathic arthritis	Serum HLA-B27
Behcet's disease	Young adults with mouth and genital ulcers and skin lesions.	HLA-B51
Coccidioidomycosis	Chorioretinitis, fever, cough; endemic along coast of California, Mexico, and South America	Serum antibodies
Cytomegalovirus	Most commonly in AIDS; severe retinitis	CMV antibody titer
Histoplasmosis (fungus)	Multiple, small, chorioretinal lesions (histo spots) (Fig. 6.137) linked to bird droppings along the Ohio and Mississippi river valleys	Histoplasmin skin test
Juvenile idiopathic arthritis	Children, fever with hepatosplenomegaly (Still's disease)	+ANA 75% of time
Lyme disease	Tick bite, skin rash, arthropathy, neurologic symptoms, mostly in New England and Mid-Atlantic states	Serum anti-borrelia burgdorferi antibodies

continued on next page

Diagnosis	Major clues	Laboratory evaluation
Lymphoma	Vitritis and anterior uveitis	MRI, lumbar puncture and/or vitreous cytology
Multiple sclerosis	Intermediate uveitis, neurologic symptoms, especially optic neuritis	MRI of brain
Polyarteritis nodosa	Systemic necrotizing vasculitis causing fatigue, myalgia, weight loss, nephritis, fever, arthralgia, iritis, keratitis, scleritis	($\uparrow$) ESR, biopsy of artery confirms diagnosis, ($\uparrow$) BUN
Reactive arthritis (Reiter's syndrome)	Iridocyclitis, urethritis, arthritis	75% (+) HLA-B27, elevated ESR, ANA
Rheumatoid arthritis	Joint pain, anemia	Rheumatoid factor +85% of time, (elevated ESR)
Sarcoidosis	Breathing disorder most common, panuveitis, lymph node enlargement	Chest x-ray, biopsy of skin, conjunctiva, lymph node, or lacrimal gl.; serum angiotensin converting enzyme (ACE)
Sjögren's syndrome	Mainly women, dry eye and mouth, arthritis	Anti-SSA/Ro and anti-SSB, subtypes of ANA
Syphylis	Retinitis, choroiditis, multitude of systemic symptoms	RPR or VDRL
Systemic lupus erythematosus	90% women, macular rash, oral and nasal ulcers, discoid lupus, arthritis, pleurisy, pericarditis	ANA is + in 95% of SLE
Toxoplasmosis (intracellular protozoa)	Very common; anterior and posterior uveitis; often in AIDS	Serum anti-toxoplasmosis gondii antibodies: 23% of US have + antibody
Toxocariasis (roundworm)	Posterior uveitis in toddlers with exposure to dog or cat	6% of US positive for serum ELISA antibodies to toxocara; eosinophilia
Tuberculosis (infects 20–43% of world population)	Cough, fever, weight loss, malaise, and sweats	Chest x-ray, PPD skin test
Wegner's granulomatosis	Systemic necrotizing granulomatous vasculitis causing uveitis and retinitis; often involves upper and lower respiratory tracts, but also kidneys and CNS. Orbital pseudotumor (p. 67) occurs in 45% of patients.	Chest x-ray shows cavitary lesions and pneumonitis; biopsy involved tissue, antineutrophil cytoplasmic antibody

Cataracts

A cataract is a cloudy lens. It should be suspected when the patient complains of blurry vision and there is a hazy view of the retina with an ophthalmoscope. The lens consists of an outside capsule surrounding a soft cortical substance and a hard inner nucleus (Fig. 6.155). The diagnosis is confirmed with a slit lamp and described the following ways:

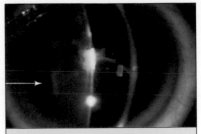

Fig. 6.157 Posterior subcapsular cataract.

1. By etiology: It is usually due to aging, but may be congenital or brought on by radiation, ultraviolet light, diabetes, trauma (especially perforation of capsule) (see Fig. 6.150) or steroids. Steroid used to treat chronic iritis in juvenile idiopathic arthritis almost always causes cataracts. There is twice the incidence in cigarette smokers. Juvenile cataracts are rare. Fifty-eight percent are idiopathic, 13% are traumatic, and 12% are inherited, most commonly in Down's syndrome. There is a long list of congenital syndromes associated with cataracts and other eye diseases. All children should have a full eye exam before age 4–5 to uncover amblyopia, but children with rare syndromes should be checked at an even earlier age, usually at the onset of the systemic symptoms.

2. By location in lens: cortex (Fig. 6.156), nucleus, or posterior subcapsule (often due to steroids (Fig. 6.157).

3. By color or pattern: The infantile inherited type is located in or around the nucleus, and often non-progressive. (Fig. 6.158).

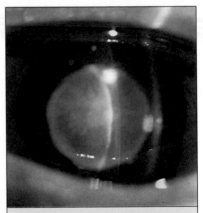

Fig. 6.158 Congenital (zonular) cataract surrounded by clear cortex.

A mature, dark brown lens is often hard and difficult to break up (Fig. 6.159) during cataract surgery.

A cataract raises two questions. Is it responsible for the decreased vision? Is it ripe? Ripe is the layman's term for whether surgery is indicated. In most cases, a surgeon waits for a reduction in vision to 20/50 or worse but indications vary with the patient's needs. Surgery is usually elective except in the case of a mature lens that might rupture or is already leaking (Fig. 6.160) or a dislocated lens in imminent danger of dropping into the vitreous or anterior chamber. Lens dislocation

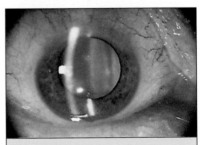

Fig. 6.159 Brunescent cataract.

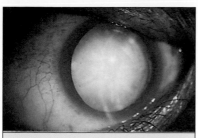

Fig. 6.160 Mature lens dislocated into the anterior chamber, obscuring pupil and iris.

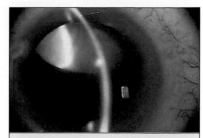

Fig. 6.161 Superiorly dislocated lens.

(Fig. 6.161) is due to rupture of the zonules. It occurs with trauma or may be associated with Marfan's disease, homocystinuria, or syphilis. Cataract surgery is performed as an outpatient procedure using local anesthesia, and is the number one major surgery performed in the US. The cornea is entered with a blade making a 3 plane incision to minimize chance of leakage and eliminate or decrease the number of sutures needed for closure (Fig. 6.162).

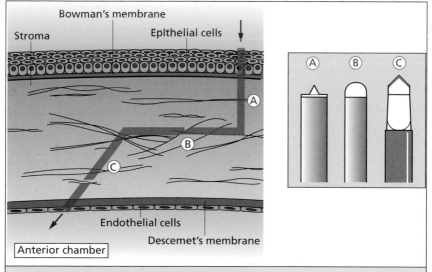

Fig. 6.162 A 3 plane corneal incision for entering the eye during cataract surgery. Blade A is guarded to create a uniform mid-depth incision approximately 3–6 mm in length. Blade B is crescent shaped for a 4 mm dissection of corneal lamellae. A downward motion with the keratome (blade C) enters the anterior chamber.

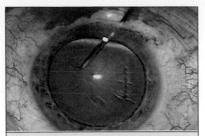

Fig. 6.163 Anterior capsulotomy: 50 punctures of anterior capsule prior to removal. Courtesy of Richard Tipperman, MD and Stephen Lichtenstein MD.

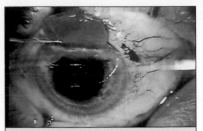

Fig. 6.164 Removal of hard nucleus in one piece. Courtesy of Richard Tipperman MD and Stephen Lichtenstein, MD.

The anterior lens capsule is then removed (Fig. 6.163). The hard nucleus is either extracted in one piece (Fig. 6.164) or liquified with a phacoemulsifier, which has a tip that vibrates 40,000 times per second (Fig. 6.165). Phaco- is a prefix referring to the lens. The advantage of phacoemulsification is that it could be done through a small wound. Its disadvantage is that it is difficult to perform and that the large amount of energy needed to emulsify a hard nucleus could damage the cornea or delicate posterior capsule.

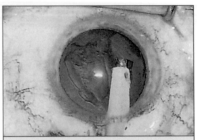

Fig. 6.165 Removal of nucleus by phacoemulsification. Courtesy of Richard Tipperman, MD and Stephen Lichtenstein, MD.

An alternative to phacoemulsification is manual phacofragmentation where a platform is placed under the hard nucleus and a chopper is placed on top. Pushing down divides the nucleus (Figs 6.166 and 6.167) into two pieces.

This technique is less expensive; requires a slightly larger wound; and gives the surgeon an option to choose a technique at which he is most skilled.

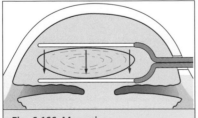

Fig. 6.166 Manual phacofragmentation of nucleus after dislocation into anterior chamber

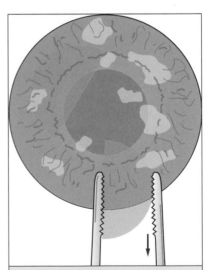

Fig. 6.167 After splitting the hard nucleus, (Fig. 6.166) it is removed in two pieces with toothed forceps. Note the white cortex still to be aspirated.

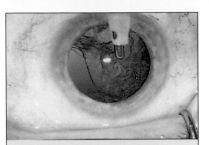

Fig. 6.168 After removing the nucleus by either technique, the surrounding cortex is removed with irrigation and aspiration. Courtesy of Richard Tipperman, MD and Stephen Lichtenstein, MD.

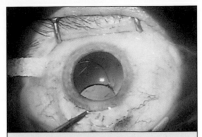

Fig. 6.169 Insertion of rigid lens through 6 mm incision. Courtesy of Richard Tipperman, MD and Stephen Lichtenstein, MD.

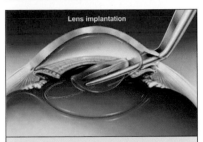

Fig. 6.170 Foldable implant inserted through 3.2 mm incision.

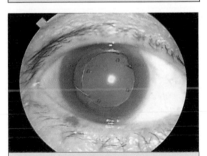

Fig. 6.171 Posterior chamber lens behind iris: preferred location.

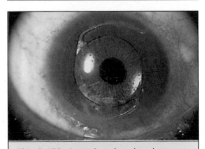

Fig. 6.172 Anterior chamber lens, sometimes used when the posterior capsule is damaged during surgery.

After the nucleus is removed by either method, the soft cortex is aspirated (Fig. 6.168) and the eye is referred to as aphakic. A spectacle lens of about +12.0 D would be required to focus the eye, but it is thick and magnifies the image 33% larger than the normal eye, so that the two eyes cannot fuse. A contact lens that magnifies the image to a lesser degree than a spectacle lens can minimize the problem of image size disparity (aniseikonia) and allow binocular vision. However, contact lenses are impractical with elderly patients. Therefore, a lens implant of about +18.0 D is inserted into the eye to restore distance vision and the eye is then referred to as pseudophakic. A-scan ultrasound is used to measure the A-P diameter of the eye. This length, together with the corneal curvature, as determined with a keratometer, gives the exact power of the intraocular lens implant needed. Intraocular lens use in infants is presently being evaluated as to its safety profile, but has gained wide acceptance after 1-2 years of age.

The lens is usually placed behind the iris (Figs 6.169–6.171), unless the posterior capsule or zonules are torn and can't support it. In these cases, it is placed in front of the iris (Fig. 6.172). This eye is now in focus for distance, but requires a spectacle for focus at near.

Multifocal lens implants that focus the eye for near and far can be used in selected patients so that they might be spectacle-free. One type has alternating rings with different refractive power (Fig. 6.173) and the other changes its refractive power by shifting its position with accommodative stimulation to the ciliary body muscle (Fig. 6.174). In eyes with significant amounts of astigmatism, a toric implant may be inserted (Fig. 6.175). Care must be taken in aligning the axis and preventing post-operative rotation.

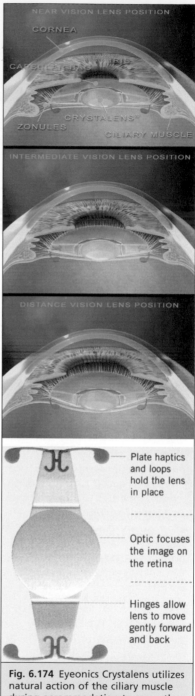

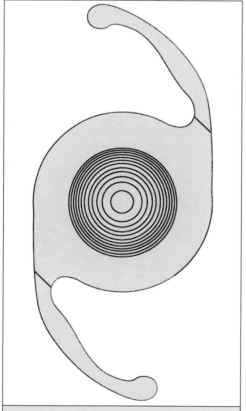

Fig. 6.173 ReSTOR multifocal intraocular lens with 12 concentric steps of focusing power which allows focus from far to near. It could cause halos and glare, especially at night.

Fig. 6.174 Eyeonics Crystalens utilizes natural action of the ciliary muscle during accommodation to move the optic of the implanted lens forward to focus for near.

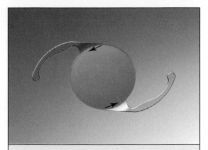

Fig. 6.175 AcrySof IQ Toric intraocular lens. A marker is first used to mark the axis of the astigmatism on the cornea of the eye. The lens is then inserted so the marks on the lens and eye line up. Image courtesy of Alcon Laboratories, Inc.

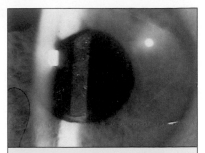

Fig. 6.176 Secondary cataract. Courtesy of Richard Tipperman MD and Stephen Lichtenstein, MD.

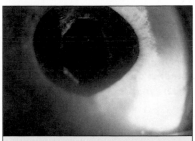

Fig. 6.177 YAG laser capsulotomy for secondary cataract of posterior capsule. Courtesy of Richard Tipperman MD and Stephen Lichtenstein, MD.

Some complications of cataract surgey

1. The posterior capsule may opacify months to years after cataract extraction in 30% of cases and is called a secondary cataract (Fig. 6.176). It may be opened with a YAG laser (Fig. 6.177)

2. If the zonules weaken, the implant could dislocate (Figs 6.178 and 6.179) in 0.3–3.0% of cases. These implants have to be supported with sutures to the iris or sclera or placed in front of the iris (Fig. 6.180)

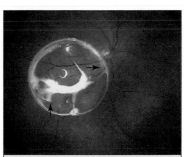

Fig. 6.179 Lens implant (↑ lens haptic) and capsular bag dislocated into the vitreous after traumatic tearing of the zonules. Courtesy of S. Parthasarethi, MD, and *Arch. Ophth.*, Sept. 2007, Vol. 125, p. 1240. Copyright 2007, Amer. Med. Assoc. All rights reserved.

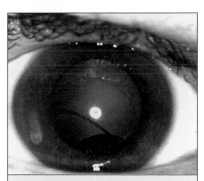

Fig. 6.178 Dislocated intraocular lens due to weakened zonules. Courtesy of Elliot Davidoff, MD.

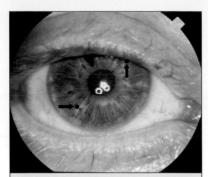

Fig. 6.180 Dislocated lens sutured to iris (↑). Courtesy of Elliot Davidoff, MD.

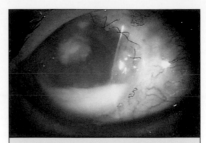

Fig. 6.181a Endophthalmitis with hypopyon following cataract surgery.

3. The corneal endothelium could be damaged resulting in corneal edema (Fig. 6.26). It is the most common reason for corneal transplant surgery

4. Retinal detachment (Fig. 7.82) occurs in 1–2% of cataract surgeries

5. Infectious endophthalmitis (Fig. 6.181a, b) is a serious complication of intraocular surgery or a penetrating intraocular injury. A culture of the aqueous and vitreous and topical, subconjunctival and intravitreal antibiotics are started immediately to save the eye and prevent blindness. Fortunately, it only occurs in 1:1000 cataract surgeries

A vitrectomy is often performed to obtain a sample for culture and to prevent formation of membranes that cause vitreo-retinal traction.

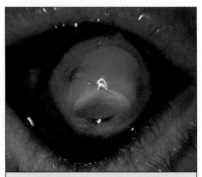

Fig. 6.181b Severe endophthalmitis with visibly dislocated lens implant in anterior chamber. Courtesy of Julia Monsonego, CRA Wills Eye Hospital.

Chapter 7
The retina and vitreous

Retinal anatomy

The retina is the sensory layer of the eye extending from the optic disk to the ora serrata (Figs 7.1–7.4).

Light stimulates the receptor cells, called rods and cones, which transmit the message to the ganglion cell on the retinal surface. The long ganglion cell axons make up the optic nerve, which synapses in the brain (Fig. 7.5a).

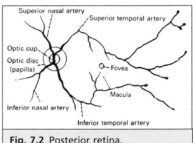

Fig. 7.1 Posterior retinal landmarks.

The macula

The macula is rich in cones and is the most sensitive area of the retina. The retinal vessels terminate at its margin, and in its center is a pit called the fovea, which produces a light reflex. The fovea has the most dense concentration of cones and is responsible for the most acute vision. This reflex decreases with age, and its absence in a young individual with a visual disturbance could indicate a macular dysfunction. When the macula is destroyed, the best corrected vision is 20/200.

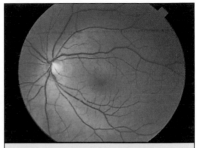

Fig. 7.2 Posterior retina.

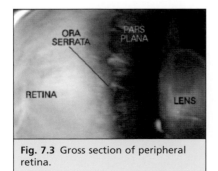

Fig. 7.3 Gross section of peripheral retina.

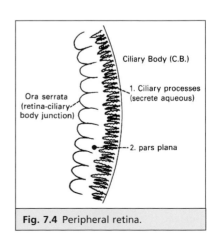

Fig. 7.4 Peripheral retina.

Manual for Eye Examination and Diagnosis, Eighth edition. Mark Leitman.
© 2012 John Wiley & Sons, Ltd. Published 2012 by John Wiley & Sons, Ltd.

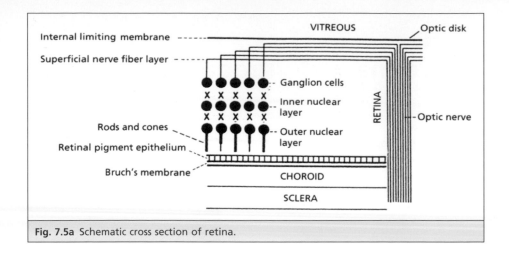

Fig. 7.5a Schematic cross section of retina.

The optic disk

The optic disk is normally orange–red with a yellow cup at its center. The retinal artery and vein pass through the optic cup and bifurcate on the surface of the disk. Proliferated retinal pigment epithelium at the disk margin is a normal finding (Fig. 7.5b).

In axial myopia, the eye is increased in length and the retina may be dragged away from the optic disk margin, exposing the sclera. This is called a myopic conus or crescent (Fig. 7.6). In extremely myopic eyes often greater than 10D, the retina is stretched so thin that it is absent in some areas, causing a loss of vision. There may be hemorrhage at the macula, called a Fuchs' spot (Fig. 7.7).

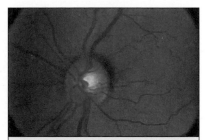

Fig. 7.5b Normal tigroid fundus with pigment around disk.

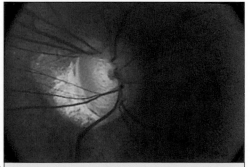

Fig. 7.6 Normal myopic conus (crescent) at disk margin.

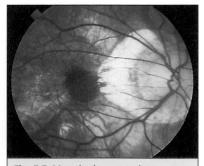

Fig. 7.7 Myopic degeneration.

Another disk variation occurs when the myelin sheath that normally covers the optic nerve extends onto the retina, appearing like white flame-shaped patches obscuring the disk margin. It is benign (Fig. 7.8). The disk margin may also be obscured by drusen (Fig. 7.9) which are small, round, translucent bodies. They may damage nerve fibers and cause an enlarged blind spot.

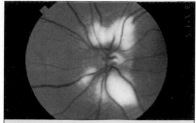

Fig. 7.8 Myelination of the optic nerve.

Fundus examination

The fundus refers to the inner part of the eye. It is evaluated with an ophthalmascope. Eye doctors usually dilate the pupils for this exam. Tropicamide (1/2–1%), which relaxes the pupillary sphincter, is preferred because of quick action (5–10 mins) and stronger effect. Phenylephrine (2.5–10%), that stimulates the dilator muscle, has a weaker effect and takes longer to act (1/2 hour). An advantage of phenylephrine is that it doesn't blur the patient as much and won't be as problematic in driving home. Both are often used together when more serious retinal disease is suspected.

The macula is examined last to minimize miosis and discomfort.

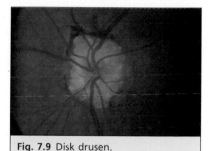

Fig. 7.9 Disk drusen.

A direct ophthalmoscope (Fig. 7.10) allows for monocular visualization of the posterior half of the fundus, where most retinal pathology is located. Use a negative lens (red) for myopic eyes, and a plus lens (black)

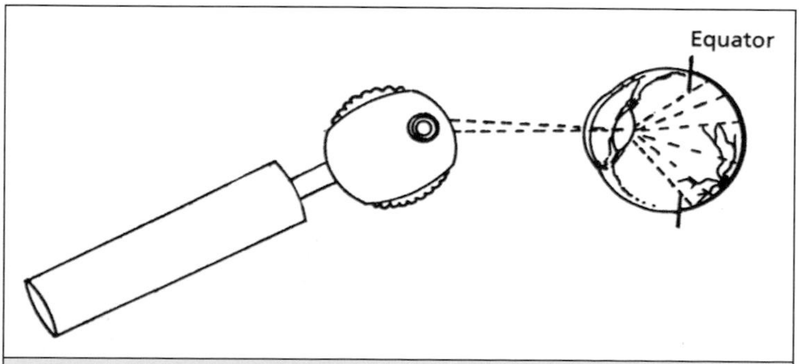

Fig. 7.10 Direct ophthalmoscope.

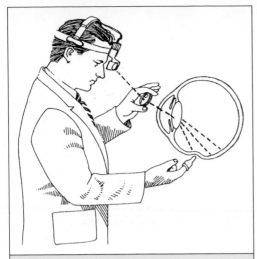

Fig. 7.11 Indirect ophthalmoscope.

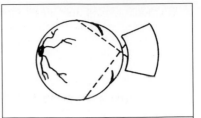

Fig. 7.12 Three-mirror contact lens.

for hyperopic eyes. Get as close to the eye as possible and minimize movement by resting your hand that is holding the ophthalmoscope on the patient's cheek, while your other hand lifts the patient's upper lid.

A binocular indirect ophthalmoscope (Fig. 7.11) consists of a light source worn over the head and a hand-held lens, which allows the entire retina to be seen in three dimensions. Retinal holes and detachments at the ora serrata can be viewed by indenting the sclera with a small thimble worn on the index finger.

A three-mirror contact lens (Fig. 7.12) used with a slit lamp gives a stereoscopic detailed view of the entire retina. It is useful in studying subtle changes in each layer of the retina, and to gauge optic cupping. Its disadvantage is the need for anesthetic drops and gelatinous a solution on the eye.

Fluorescein angiography

(Figs 7.13 and 7.14)

Fluorescein dye is injected intravenously. As it passes through the retinal circulation, fundus photographs are made in a rapid sequence. This test is useful for evaluating retinal

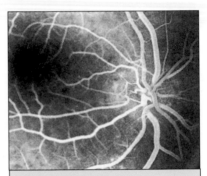

Fig. 7.13 Normal fluorescein angiogram.

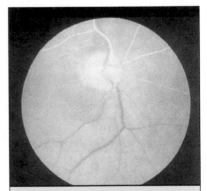

Fig. 7.14 Fluorescein angiogram of inferior retinal artery occlusion showing lack of perfusion inferiorly after 15.4 seconds.

circulation. It demonstrates rate of flow, leakage from capillaries, staining of tissues, areas of nonperfusion, and neovascularization. Retinal blood vessels do not normally leak.

Papilledema (choked disk)

(Figs 7.15 and 7.16)

Papilledema is swelling of the optic nerve specifically due to elevated intracranial pressure that causes a reduction in the ability of fluid to exit the eye. It is always serious. The intraocular congestion results in a swollen, elevated optic disc with blurred margins. As it progresses, veins become engorged and flame-shaped hemorrhages and cotton-wool spots develop in the peripapillary area.

In 80% of normal eyes, there are subtle pulsations of the retinal veins as they exit from the globe at the optic cup. If pulsations are not visible, they can almost always be elicited by exerting slight pressure on the globe (through the lid). In papilledema, one cannot see spontaneous or elicited venous pulsations. Swelling of the optic disk damages the surrounding retina and enlarges the blind spot, which helps confirm the diagnosis (Fig. 7.17) and is helpful in monitoring the progression of the disease. The elevated intracranial pressure often causes headache, confusion, nausea, and visual obscurations. Diplopia occurs if the pressure compromises the sixth cranial nerve. Prolonged increased pressure can permanently damage the brain

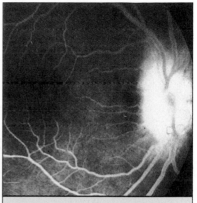

Fig. 7.15 Fluorescein angiogram of papilledema with leakage of dye from disk.

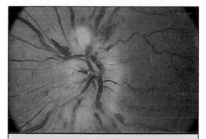

Fig. 7.16 Papilledema with elevated disk, engorged veins, and flame-shaped hemorrhages.

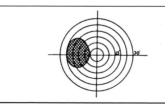

Fig. 7.17 An enlarged blind spot can be plotted most accurately on a tangent screen. Visual field testing of the size of the blind spot and contraction of the peripheral field must be monitored closely since this is often the only way to know how the disease is being controlled, since spinal tap pressures are dangerous and not that reliable.

and optic nerve. Common causes are side effect of drugs, such as tetracycline, vitamin A toxicity, and retinoids used to treat severe acne and psoriasis. Brain tumors, hemorrhages, and infections also could elevate intracranial pressure.

Idiopathic intracranial hypertension (pseudotumor cerebri) is a condition with elevated pressure that has no obvious cause. It often occurs in young, overweight women and is first discovered during a routine eye exam that reveals papilledema. Treatment of these women includes weight loss, oral Diamox (acetazolamide), and a low-sodium diet. If unsuccessful, then surgical optic nerve sheath fenestration or ventriculoperitoneal shunting could be tried.

Pseudopapilledema

There are many conditions that can mimic the optic disk changes of papilledema and every clue must be considered.

A swollen disk caused by optic neuritis (see Fig. 3.39), is associated with a Marcus Gunn pupil and loss of central vision, whereas in early papilledema, the pupil is normal and there is usually no loss of visual acuity unless edema extends to the macula (Fig. 7.18) or optic atrophy has already occurred.

Early papilledema may be difficult to distinguish from drusen of the disk (Fig. 7.9) and myelinated nerve fibers (Fig. 7.8). All three blur the margin and cause an enlarged blind spot (Fig. 7.17). On fluorescein-angiography, however, only papilledema has leakage of dye

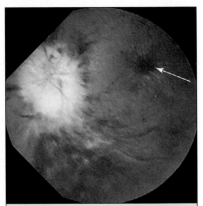

Fig. 7.18 Papilledema with macular star (↑) due to vitamin A toxicity.

(Fig. 7.15). A hyperopic eye might have a small disk with blurred margin, but there is no leakage with fluorescein angiography. Like papilledema, central retinal vein occlusion (Fig. 7.38) may have venous engorgement, a blurred disk margin, and cotton-wool spots. But in central retinal vein occlusion, the flame hemorrhages extend out to the periphery and there is more loss of vision. Malignant systemic hypertension (BP 220/120 mmHg) also causes a papilledema-like retinal appearance, which is easily distinguished by measuring blood pressure on all patients with blurry disk margins (Fig. 7.22). Orbital diseases decreasing venous outflow from the eye can cause swelling of the disk. Causes include orbital tumors and infections. Idiopathic inflammation of the orbit, also called orbital pseudotumor, (Fig. 5.9), must be considered. Don't confuse orbital pseudotumor, which does not cause papilledema, with previously discussed pseudotumor cerebri, which does. In these orbital diseases, one looks for localizing signs, such as proptosis. Cavernous sinus disease can also obstruct venous drainage (Fig. 3.60).

Retinal Blood Vessels

Retinal vessel walls are normally transparent. They are visualized because of the blood within them. In arteriosclerosis, as the vessel walls become hyalinized, they develop a white reflex.

The vessel walls may also whiten when inflamed in conditions such as systemic lupus erythematosus (Fig. 1.4), sarcoidosis (Fig. 6.135), cytomegalovirus infection (Fig. 6.147), sickle cell disease and trait (Fig. 7.20). The damaged vessel may eventually develop a permanent white sheath and a thread-like lumen. Loss of blood flow, as occurs in renal artery occlusion, may also cause this change (Fig. 7.30).

Abnormal capillaries may grow inside the eye in a misguided response to ischemia from retinal artery or vein occlusion and proliferative diabetic retinopathy (see book cover).

They are due to liberation of vascular endothelial growth factor (VEGF). Panretinal laser photocoagulation may be used to destroy large areas of the hypoxic retina thus decreasing the secretion of VEGF. A total of 1,500 burns is administered to each eye in 2 sessions (Fig. 7.19).

The biggest breakthroughs in ophthalmology in recent years are anti-VEGF drugs, ranibuzumob (Lucentis), and bevacizumab (Avastin), which, when injected into the vitreous, causes regression of these abnormal vessels. It is now being used as a first-line, treatment of wet macular degeneration and for macular edema due to retinal vein occlusions and diabetic retinopathy.

Sickle cell hemoglobinopathy leads to red cells taking on a sickle shape in deoxygenated blood (Fig. 7.20). Sickle cell trait (HbAS) affects 8% of African Americans, with 0.4% having sickle cell disease (HbSS) and 0.2% having HbSC disease. Retinal neovascularization resembling "seafans" (Fig. 7.21) occur at the edge of infarcted (pale) areas. Confirm with a sickle cell prep where a deoxygenating agent is added to a patient's blood. It's positive if RBCs assume a crescent (sickle) shape.

Fig. 7.19 Panretinal photocoagulation (PRP) uses an argon laser to apply 1500 burns to partially destroy retinal tissue while carefully avoiding the central fovea. Courtesy Daniel Roth, MD.

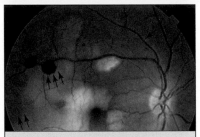

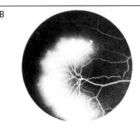

Fig. 7.20 Sickle cell retinopathy with vascular inflammation (↑), pale areas of ischemic retina salmon patch intraretinal haemorrhages (↑↑) and pre-retinal haemorrhages (↑↑↑). This occurred in a 26 year-old black male presenting to the emergency department with an acute MI, renal failure, and cholecystitis.

A

B

Fig. 7.21A Sickle cell retinopathy with compensatory neovascularization at edge of infarcted retina.

Fig. 7.21B Fluorescein angiogram with leakage from abnormal new vessels.

Reprinted with permission from SLACK, Inc., Cohen, S.B., Greenberg, M., Fletcher, M.E. & Jednock, N.J. (1986). Diagnosis & Management of Ocular Complications of Sickle Cell Hemoglobin Retinopathy, *Ophthalmic Surgery*, 17(2), 110–116.

Hypertensive retinopathy

At their junctions, the arteries and veins share a common sheath. As the arteriole wall thickens (arteriosclerosis), it takes on a silvery appearance and causes indentation of the venule, referred to as A-V nicking (Fig. 7.23), This can lead to a retinal vein occlusion.

Blood Pressure	
Normal	< 120/80
Pre-hypertension	120–139/80–89
Hypertension	>140/90

It was shown in a large 20 year study that half of those treated for hypertension in the US failed to be controlled at 140/90 as recommended.

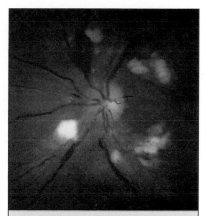

Fig. 7.22 Stage III hypertensive retinopathy with cotton-wool spots, flame-shaped hemorrhages, and narrowing.

Retinal vein occlusion

Retinal vein occlusions cause a painless decrease in vision with haemorrhages extending to the peripheral retina (Fig. 7.38). Acutely, there are flame-shaped hemorrhages (Fig. 7.24 and 7.25) and dot and blot haemorrhages which may last for years. Cotton-wool spots and a poorly reactive pupil usually indicate an ischemic retina and is more ominous. Ischemia is confirmed with fluorescein angiography. One half of the ischemic cases stimulate secretion of vascular endothelial growth factor

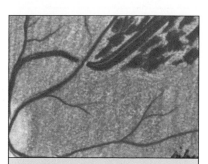

Fig. 7.23 Drawing of branch retinal vein occlusion with flame hemorrhages and A-V nicking. As the arteriole wall thickens, the A-V crossings change from an acute to a right angle.

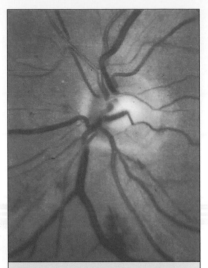

Fig. 7.24 Arteriosclerosis with partial vein occlusion demonstrated by engorged vein inferiorly and a secondary flame hemorrhage. "Silver wire" changes are noted at the superior disk margin and irregular narrowing of the artery is noted on the left superior side of the figure.

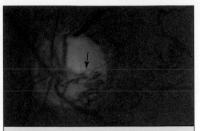

Fig. 7.25 Central retinal vein occlusion 3 months after occurrence. Collateral curlicue vessels on disc and retina (↑) help venous blood exit the eye. They don't bleed or leak fluorescein as do new blood vessels in diabetes (cover of book). Courtesy of Julia Monsonego, CRA Wills Eye Hospital.

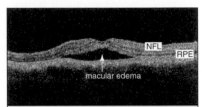

Fig. 7.26 OCT of retinal macular edema after retinal vein occlusion. RPE, retinal pigment epithelium; NFL, nerve fiber layer. An OCT reveals structural changes of the retina as compared with fluorescein angiography which shows abnormalities in blood flow.

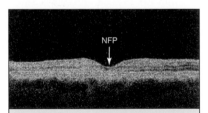

Fig. 7.27 OCT of resolved macular edema from retinal vein occlusion after intravitreal triamcinolone injection. Vision improved from 20/400 to 20/30. NFP, normal foveal pit. Courtesy of Jennifer Hancock.

(VEGF) causing new blood vessel growth on the iris which could leak, bleed, and lead to glaucoma. Not all new vessels are bad. Late onset, tortuous retino-choroidal collateral vessels could develop on the optic disk, and elsewhere on the retina, and are beneficial in helping the obstructed venous blood exit the eye via the choroidal route (Fig. 7.25). If macular edema occurs, it may be treated with localized laser to the retina, intravitreal Lucentis (anti-VEGF), or intravitreal steroid injection. There are corticosteroid intravitreal implants that provide a prolonged, slow release.

Optical coherence tomography (OCT) is a new technology to obtain high-resolution cross-section images of the eye. It is analogous to ultrasound except it uses light instead of sound. It is especially useful to monitor macular edema (Figs 7.26 and 7.27) and macular holes (Figs 7.88 and 7.89).

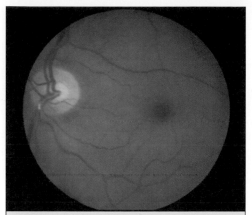

Fig. 7.28 Retinal artery occlusion with a cholesterol Hollenhorst plaque on disk and a cherry-red macula.

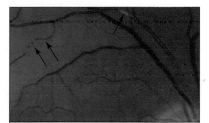

Fig. 7.29 Branch retinal artery occlusion with embolus (↑) and sludging of blood (box-car effect ↑↑) due to a decreased flow. Courtesy of Julia Monsonego, CRA Wilis Eye Hospital.

Retinal artery occlusion

Retinal artery occlusion (Figs 7.28 and 7.29) causes sudden loss of vision. Carotid artery plaques (see Fig. p.155) or heart disease such as arrhythmias, endocarditis, or valve disease may liberate fine platelets or larger cholesterol emboli (Hollenhorst plaque), which lodge in arterial bifurcations. Sludging of blood flow gives a box-car appearance (Fig. 7.29). Some irreparable loss of vision usually occurs within 1 hour, and the loss is almost impossible to reverse after 12 hours. Eventually optic atrophy results (Fig. 7.30). Any treatment is of questionable value. You could have patient breathe into a paper bag to elevate CO_2 which dilates the artery; lower eye pressure with oral or topical medications; gently massage the eye to get embolus to move on. Call eye doctor immediately to tap anterior chamber which further lowers eye pressure.

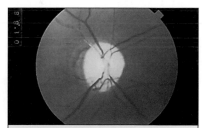

Fig. 7.30 Late-stage retinal artery occlusion with optic atrophy and arteries that are thread-like and sheathed.

Diabetic retinopathy (front cover)

Type 1 diabetes (insulin dependent) is due to decreased secretion of insulin by the B-cells in the pancreas and is largely caused by an autoimmune process. Type 2 diabetes (adult onset) is primarily due to cellular resistance to insulin. Type 2 accounts for 90% of diabetes and its cause is strongly related to obesity and lack of exercise. Both types cause elevated blood sugar with damage to the microvasculature of the retina. Twenty-five percent of eyes have changes after 10 years, 50% after 15 years, and 80% after 20 years.

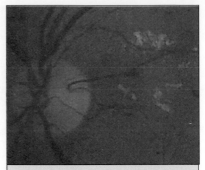

Fig. 7.31 Stage 1. Background retinopathy with microaneurysms, exudates, and dot hemorrhages.

There are three progressive stages of diabetic retinopathy:

1 Non-proliferative or background retinopathy initially presents with microaneurysms (Figs 7.31 and 7.32). These may leak and cause edema, proteinaceous exudates, and dot hemorrhages at the macula. This is the most common reason for loss of vision in diabetic retinopathy. The macular edema is usually treated with focal laser photocoagulation. If unsuccessful, one may try intravitreal triamcinolone (steroid) injections, vitrectomy surgery, or an injection of intravitreal anti-vascular endothelial growth factor.

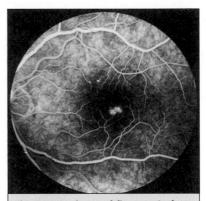

Fig. 7.32 Leakage of fluorescein from microaneurysms. Normal retinal vessels do not leak.

2 Preproliferatlve retinopathy (Fig. 7.33) is due to widespread capillary closure (Fig. 7.34) causing retinal ischemia. There are cotton wool

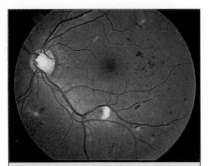

Fig. 7.33 Stage 2. Preproliferative retinopathy with cotton-wool spots, microaneurysms, and dot hemorrhages.

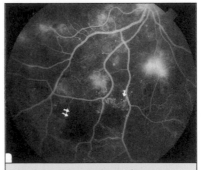

Fig. 7.34 Fluorescein angiogram showing neovascularization (↓) adjacent to dark area of capillary nonperfusion (↓↓).

spots, venous beading, blot hemorrhages, and the absence of blood flow on fluorescein angiography.

3 Proliferative diabetic retinopathy occurs when the ischemic areas of the retina stimulate the growth of abnormal curlicue capillaries on or around the disk (Fig. 7.35) and the iris. The former may bleed into the vitreous totally obstructing vision and a view of the retina. They then can cause fibrotic membranes (Fig. 7.36) that contract resulting in retinal detachments. Panretinal photocoagulation destroys part of the ischemic retina, thus reducing the release of VEGF that causes neovascularization (Fig. 7.19). Intravitreal injection of anti-VEGF causes regression of new vessels, but it's not as yet routinely used. This third stage often occurs late in the course of diabetes and is associated with other serious systemic vascular diseases and an associated 56% 5-year survival rate. All diabetics should see an eye doctor yearly for a retina examination through a dilated pupil.

To minimize these changes, one should ideally keep the fasting blood sugar less than 110 mg/dL, blood pressure less than 130/80, exercise, stay thin, reduce abdominal obesity, and keep blood glycosylated hemoglobin (HbAlc) levels less than 6.5%, although 6.0% is even better. HbAlc gives an estimate of the preceding 3 month control of blood sugar. For each additional percentage point of HbA1c, there is a 50% increase in complications of diabetes. By lowering systolic BP 10 mg/Hg, there could be

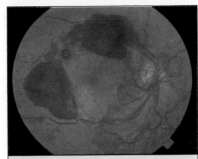

Fig. 7.35 Stage 3a. Proliferative retinopathy with neovascularization and preretinal hemorrhages.

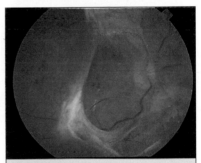

Fig. 7.36 Stage 3b. Fibrous proliferation. These membranes may contract and cause a retinal detachment.

Approximate Equivalent	
HbA1c (%)	Mean non-fasting glucose (mg/dL)
4	65
5	100
6	135
7	170
8	205
9.5	226
10.0	240
10.5	255
11.0	269
11.5	283

Depth of retinal hemorrhages

Preretinal hemorrhages

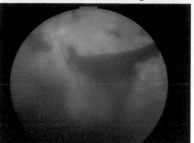

Fig. 7.37 Preretinal hemorrhages lie between the retinal internal limiting membrane and the posterior hyaloid surface of the vitreous. They may layer out to a boat shape. Common causes include proliferative diabetic retinopathy, trauma, vitreous detachments and leukemia (Fig. 7.42). This blood could break into the vitreous and obscure the view.

Superficial hemorrhages

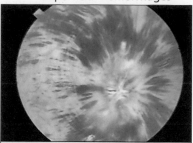

Fig. 7.38 The central retinal vein occlusion (CRVO) above shows superficial flame-shaped hemorrhages that follow the contour of the nerve fiber layer and radiate from the optic disk far out into the periphery. Flame hemorrhages also occur in papilledema, diabetes, hypertension, and optic neuritis, but don't extend to the peripheral retina as in CRVO.

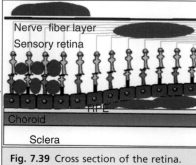

Nerve fiber layer

Sensory retina

RPE

Choroid

Sclera

Fig. 7.39 Cross section of the retina.

Deep retinal hemorrhages

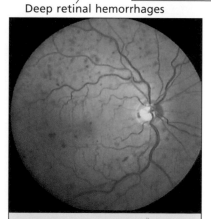

Fig. 7.40 Intraretinal hemorrhages in partial central retinal vein occlusion. Dot and blot hemorrhages occur most often in diabetes and retinal vein occlusion.

Subretinal hemorrhages

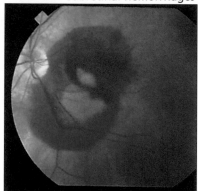

Fig. 7.41 Wet macular degeneration with subretinal hemorrhages that are grayish in appearance since they are under the retinal pigment epithelium (RPE). The red hemorrhages broke into the deep retina.

a 40% reduction in retinopathy. A small number of non-diabetics may also develop a mild form of retinopathy resembling diabetic retinopathy indicating that there may be factors other than fasting plasma glucose levels responsible for these changes.

Age-related macular degeneration (AMD)

Age related macular degeneration (AMD) occurs after age 50 and is the leading cause of blindness in elderly persons. Twenty-five percent of 70 year old persons have signs of the condition, and this number increases to 50% by age 90. The main symptom is loss of central vision. In a normal retina (Fig. 7.43), the retinal pigment epithelium (RPE) has tight junctions protecting the sensory retina from leakage of more permeable choroidal capillaries. The RPE also metabolically supports the rods and cones and creates an adhesive force with the overlying neurosensory retina, which prevents retinal detachments. There are two types of AMD. The more common dry non-neovascular type accounts for 90% of cases. In dry AMD, Bruch's membrane degenerates by fragmenting in some areas and thickening with hyaline (drusen) in other areas (Figs 7.44–7.45, 7.59). There is often

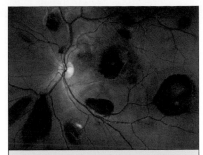

Fig. 7.42 White centered preretinal hemorrhages called Roth spots may occur in anemia, leukemia, and in bacterial endocarditis. Courtesy of Debra Brown: COT, CRA Univ. of San Francisco.

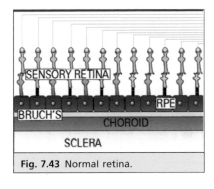

Fig. 7.43 Normal retina.

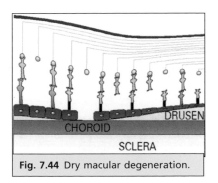

Fig. 7.44 Dry macular degeneration.

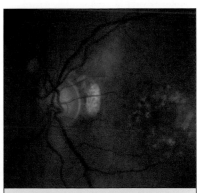

Fig. 7.45 Dry, atrophic macular degeneration with pigment, mottling, drusen, and loss of the foveal reflex. Courtesy of Elliot Davidoff, MD.

pigment mottling and loss of the foveal reflex. The RPE on top of the drusen degenerates. The overlying sensory retina metabolically dependent on the RPE thins out, resulting in atrophic macular degeneration. If enough retina disappears, the underlying choroidal vasculature is easily visualized with an ophthalmoscope. Advanced dry macular degeneration is termed geographic atrophy (Fig. 7.46) because of the large circumscribed atrophic areas through which choroidal vessels can be seen.

Dry macular degeneration may be treated with supplements of vitamins A, E, C, zinc, lutein, zeaxanthin, and omega-3 fatty acids. These are available in various combinations over-the-counter. These supplements reduce loss of vision by 25%. Avoiding cigarettes and wearing UV protective lenses are also beneficial.

About 10% of the dry-type degeneration may progress to the wet-type in which choroidal blood vessels (subretinal neovascularization) penetrate the damaged Bruch's membrane (Figs 7.40 and 7.41). These vessels may bleed, causing a hemorrhagic detachment of the RPE, which appears dark red. When it breaks into the sensory retina, it appears bright red (Fig. 7.48). Eventually, the blood could fibrose and form a white scar (Fig. 7.50) called disciform macular degeneration. A fluorescein

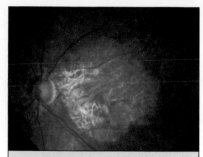

Fig. 7.46 The advanced stage of dry macular degeneration is called geographic (AMD). The thinned retina exposes underlying choroidal vasculatlure. Courtesy of Elliot Davidoff, MD.

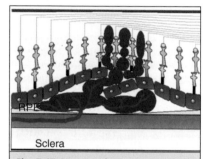

Fig. 7.47 Neovascular age-related macular degeneration.

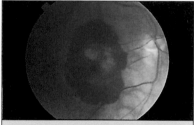

Fig. 7.48 Hemorrhagic stage of macular degeneration.

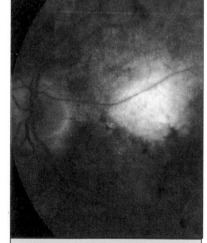

Fig. 7.49 Fluorescein angiogram of subretinal neovascular membrane.

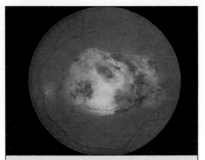

Fig. 7.50 Late stage disciform scar. Courtesy of Leo Masciulli.

angiogram may reveal subretinal vessels before they bleed (Fig. 7.49). An early symptom of progression from the dry to wet form may be that straight lines become wavy on the Amsler grid. The patient may monitor at home (Fig. 3.48 and appendix).

The treatment for wet macular degeneration is monthly intravitreal injections of Lucentis (ranibizumab) (Fig. 7.51) for an as yet undetermined number of months. This drug antagonizes vascular endothelial growth factor (VEGF) causing regression of abnormal vessels.

If anti-VEGF therapy is not effective, laser photodynamic therapy may be used. Intravenously administered verteprofin (Visudyne) concentrates in the choroidal vasculature. A low-energy laser is then aimed at the vessels, activating the dye, causing most cell death inside the vessel, but also some collateral retinal damage. Intravitreal steroid (triamcinolone) injection may be added to reduce inflammation.

The remaining 10% of macular degenerations are due to juvenile inherited types, chorioretinitis, infection, and staring at the sun. Reassure patients that they never go totally blind, but only lose central vision, often resulting in 20/400 vision.

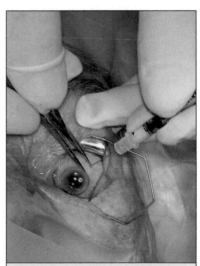

Fig. 7.51 Pars plana injection of anti-VEGF Lucentis to treat wet age-related macular degeneration. Calipers measure site 3.5 mm posterior to limbus. Courtesy of Elliot Davidoff, MD.

Central serous retinopathy

This is a macular disease in which a defect in the RPE allows choroidal fluid to leak into the sensory retina (Figs 7.52–7.54). It usually affects males aged 25–40 and may be triggered by corticosteroids and stress. Symptoms are decreased and distorted vision. Wavy lines are demonstrated with an Amsler grid. Ophthalmoscopically, it is difficult to visualize the clear, oval elevation of the retina. Eighty to ninety percent clear within a few months. Laser photocoagulation may be used if leakage continues for 6 months.

Pseudoxanthoma elasticum is a systemic disease. There may be cardiovascular abnormalities, gastrointestinal hemorrhages, and loose skin folds on the neck (Fig. 7.60b). On fundus exam, there are angioid streaks (Fig. 7.60a). Angioid streaks also occur in Ehlers–Danlos, Paget's, and sickle cell disease.

Albinism

Albinism has many forms and refers to inherited hypopigmentation. Common findings in all types involving the eye are photophobia, hypopigmentation of the retina (Fig. 7.61) and transillumination of the iris with a penlight at the limbus (Fig. 7.62). Additional findings may include nystagmus, a hypoplastic macula with absence of a foveal reflex, reduced vision, refractive errors, decreased immunity, and decreased pigmentation of the hair and skin (Fig. 7.63).

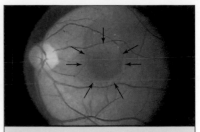

Fig. 7.52 Central serous retinopathy.

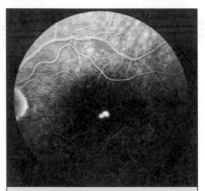

Fig. 7.53 Fluorescein leakage through the RPE in central serous retinopathy.

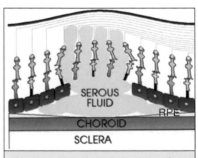

Fig. 7.54 Central serous retinopathy.

White and yellow retinal lesions

Cotton-wool spots

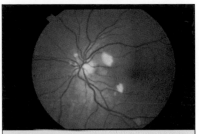

Fig. 7.55 Cotton-wool spots in AIDS. Precapillary arteriolar closure causes infarctions of the superficial nerve fiber layer. These white, cloud-like lesions cluster around the disk and obscure the underlying retina.

Inflammatory cells

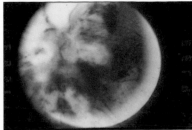

Fig. 7.56 White, inflammatory cells in cytomegalovirus retinitis. Courtesy of Joseph Walsh, MD, Chairman, NY Medical College and NY Eye and Ear Hospital.

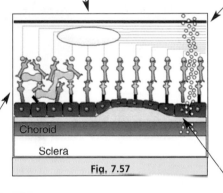

Choroid

Sclera

Fig. 7.57

Hard (waxy) exudate

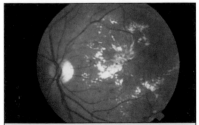

Fig. 7.58 Exudate in background diabetic retinopathy. Leaking fluid from vessels leaves behind an irregularly shaped waxy, yellowish, lipoprotein residue. It is seen most often in diabetes and retinal vein occlusions.

Retinal drusen

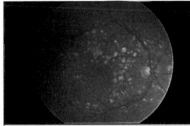

Fig. 7.59 Drusen in early macular degeneration due to thickening of Bruch's membrane and degeneration of overlying retinal pigment epithelium. Drusen are dull, white, round, often bilateral, and uniformly distributed. They are sometimes hard to distinguish from waxy exudates that are yellow and irregular in shape and distribution.

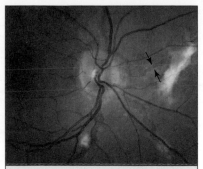

Fig. 7.60a Pseudoxanthoma elasticum: Angioid streaks are breaks in Bruch's membrane (↑) that radiate from the peripapillary area. Courtesy of Julia Monsonego, CRA Wills Eye Hospital.

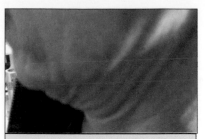

Fig. 7.60b Don't confuse pseudoxanthoma elasticum and Ehlers–Danlos (E.D.) syndrome. Both are inherited diseases of skin elasticity (loose skin on the neck), arterial aneurysms, blue sclera, and retinal angioid streaks. Unique to E.D. is hyperextensibility of the joints.

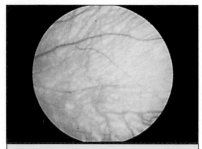

Fig. 7.61 Albinotic fundus.

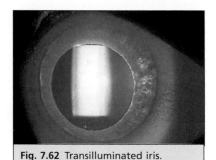

Fig. 7.62 Transilluminated iris.

Retinitis pigmentosa (Figs 7.64–7.67)

This is a slowly progressive hereditary rod–cone degeneration. Inheritance patterns include autosomal dominant or recessive and x-linked recessive. Since it begins in the retinal periphery, the fIrst loss is peripheral

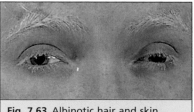

Fig. 7.63 Albinotic hair and skin.

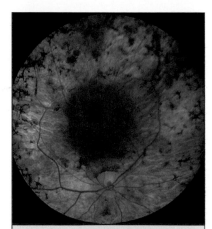

Fig. 7.64 Retinitis pigmentosa with boney pigmented spicules. Courtesy of John Fingert, MD and Arch. of Ophth., Sept 2008, Vol. 126, No. 9, p. 1301–1303.

and night vision (Fig. 7.66), often sparing central visual acuity for many years. The retina has pigmentary changes resembling bone corpuscles. The diagnosis is confirmed with an electroretinogram.

At least three separate researchers have restored some vision in humans with implantation of silicon microchips in the subretinal space which convert light energy into electrical current (Fig. 7.67).

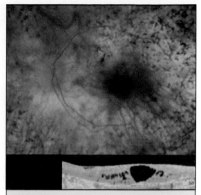

Fig. 7.65 Retinitis pigmentosa with macular cyst clearly visible on OCT. Courtesy of Alexis Smith, CRA, OCT-C Kellogg Eye Center, Ann Arbor, MI.

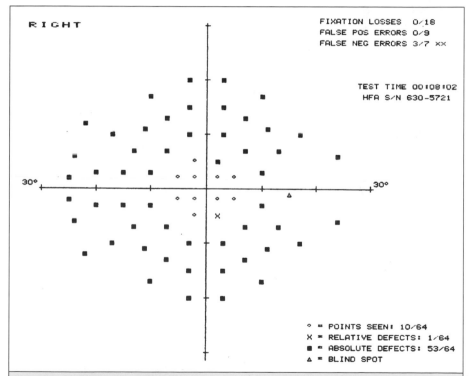

Fig. 7.66 Constricted visual field in late-stage retinitis pigmentosa. Dark squares indicate absence of vision.

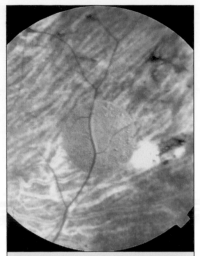

Fig. 7.67 Silicone microchip in the subretinal space. Note black pigment clumping typical of retinitis pigmentosa. Courtesy of Alan and Vincent Chow.

Retinoblastoma (Figs 7.68 and 7.69)

This is a malignant tumor of the retina often appearing by 2 years of age. Most occur from a genetic mutation that survivors may transmit as a mendelian dominant. There may be one or more white, elevated retinal masses which are bilateral 30% of the time. A CT scan often reveals calcifications in the tumor. Removal of the eye is indicated for unilateral cases. When both eyes are involved, the worse eye may be enucleated and the other treated with chemo-, radio-, laser-, or cryotherapy. All infants at 3 and 6 months should be tested for a red pupillary reflex. An ophthalmoscope light reveal symmetric red reflections with no opacities.

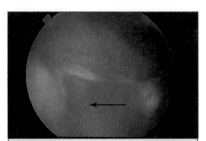

Fig. 7.68 Retinoblastoma. Courtesy of David Taylor.

Retinopathy of prematurity (ROP)

This disease of newborns occurs in premature infants weighing less than 2000 grams or having a gestational age of 28 weeks or less. It occurs more often when oxygen was administered.

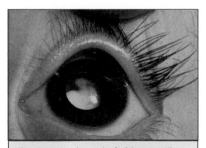

Fig. 7.69 Leukocoria (white pupil) due to retinoblastoma.

Normal vascularization of the retina progresses peripherally and is not normally completed until 1 month after birth. Oxygen given to newborns stops this normal vascularization process. When the oxygen is discontinued, the avascular peripheral retina stimulates new vessel growth (Figs 7.70 and 7.71). These new vessels, however, are now abnormal and may bleed, resulting in vitreous hemorrhage with fibrous proliferation. It could drag the retina (Fig. 7.72), sometimes causing a retinal detachment. The ideal therapy is comprehensive prenatal care to reduce the number of premature births and careful monitoring of oxygen in the nursery.

Unfortunately, ROP is becoming more prevalent because of advances in neonatal intensive care units causing an improvement in survival for very low birthweight infants. An eye doctor should check the peripheral retina at 6 weeks of chronological age or 32 weeks gestational age, whichever was earlier.

Laser photocoagulation, or less often transscleral cryotherapy, may be used to scar the avascular retina in stage 3 when the demarcation line is elevated with fibrovascular proliferation. Rigid examination and treatment guidelines and frequent poor visual outcomes are causing a shortage of doctors willing to follow these infants and be exposed to high cost litigation. A web-based telemedicine system is presently being evaluated. Retinal photographs taken by nurses and technicians are being sent to remote sites to be reviewed by experts.

Vitreous

The vitreous is a clear gel made up of collagen fibrils that fills the interior of the globe like air fills a balloon.

Disorders in the vitreous often cause debris to be deposited in this clear gel. The patient perceives the changes as shifting floaters. A recent onset of this symptom requires a dilated retina examination with an indirect ophthalmoscope.

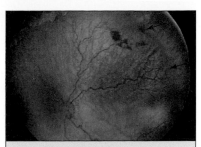

Fig. 7.70 Stage 3 retinopathy of prematurity (ROP). Note line of demarcation where normal retinal vessels stopped growing (↑). It is initially a flat line (Stage 1) then it forms a ridge (Stage 2) before abnormal vessels start growing (Stage 3). Laser treatment will hopefully prevent a Stage 4 retinal detachment.

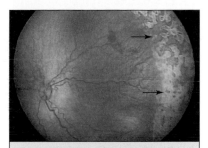

Fig. 7.71 Regression of abnormal vessels and hemorrhages after treating ischemic peripheral retina with laser (↑). Courtesy of Anna L. Ellis, MD and *Arch. Ophth.*, Oct. 2002, Vol. 120, p. 1405. Copyright 2002, Amer. Med. Assoc. All rights reserved.

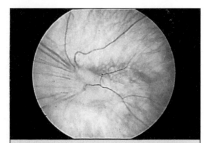

Fig. 7.72 Late stage of retinopathy of prematurity with disk and retinal vessels dragged peripherally.

White cells in the vitreous (Fig. 7.73) are found in uveitis, endophthalmitis, or papillitis. Red cells are seen in vitreous hemorrhages, which occur most often often with diabetic retinopathy. Retinal holes, detachments, and trauma are less common causes (Figs. 7.75, 7.81 and 7.82).

In asteroid hyalosis, hundreds of small, spherical balls are suspended in the vitreous and, amazingly, aren't very annoying to the patient. When questioned, they admit to seeing floaters (Fig. 7.76). These calcium phospholipid crystals deposit in the vitreous for no apparent reason. Ophthalmoscopically, these appear like stars in the galaxy and are benign, requiring no treatment. If there is haziness of the vitreous, cornea, or lens to sufficiently obscure the view of the retina, a B-scan ultrasound can be ordered (Fig. 7.74).

Posterior vitreous detachment (PVD)

The vitreous normally liquefies and shrinks with age with a prevalence of 63% in people over 70. It is most strongly adherent to the retina at the vitreous base (near the ora serrata), the macula, and the optic disc. Traction on these areas can normally cause some flashing lights and floaters with no consequences. However, the PVD could tear the very

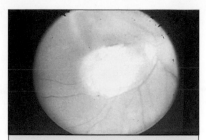

Fig. 7.73 Hazy view of toxoplasmosis choroiditis due to white cells in the vitreous.

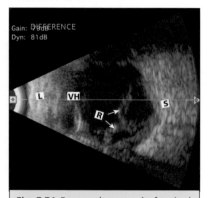

Fig. 7.74 B-scan ultrasound of retinal detachment (R) with vitreous hemorrhage (VH), posterior surface of lens (L), and sclera (S).

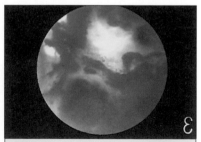

Fig. 7.75 Blunt trauma, causing pre-, intra-, and subretinal hemorrhage is referred to as commotio retinae. Hemorrhage may extend into the vitreous. Traumatic hemorrhages also occur in 85% of cases of Shaken-Baby syndrome and must be looked for when physical abuse is suspected.

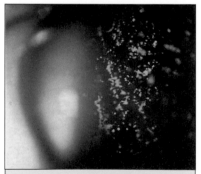

Fig. 7.76 Slit lamp view of asteroid hyalosis, with lens seen on left and vitreous on right.

thin superficial internal limiting membrane (ILM) covering the nerve fiber layer of the retina.

Breaks in the ILM allow glial cells to grow onto the surface of the retina. This gliosis at first is a clear, glistening cellophane-appearing membrane which can then progress to a more translucent and then opaque epiretinal membrane (ERM) that can reduce vision. This ERM can contract and cause macular pucker with wrinkling of the retina and distortion of vision (Fig. 7.78). If vision is significantly affected, a surgical vitrectomy and membranectomy can be performed (Fig. 7.79).

In 12% of cases of PVD, the tear is more severe than just the ILM and extends through the sensory retina. Of these retinal holes, 40% going on to develop a retinal detachment (Figs 7.80–7.84).

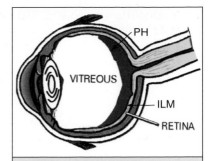

Fig. 7.77 Posterior vitreous detachment. The posterior surface of the vitreous is called the posterior hyaloid (PH). The membrane covering the retinal surface is called the internal limiting membrane (ILM).

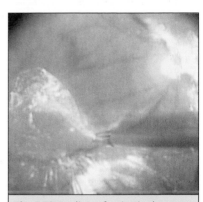

Fig. 7.79 Peeling of epiretinal membrane. Reprinted from *Amer. J. Ophth.*, Sept. 2009, Vol. 148/3, p. 338. Dyes in Ocular Surgery, Michel Eid Parah, Maurkio Maia, Eduardo B. Rodrigues with permission from Elsevier.

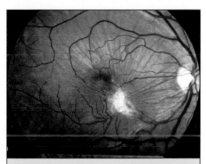

Fig. 7.78 Macular pucker occurs in 6% of the population. Courtesy of Jennifer Hancock.

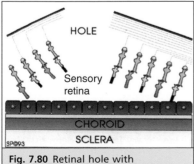

Fig. 7.80 Retinal hole with detachment of sensory retina from pigment epithelium.

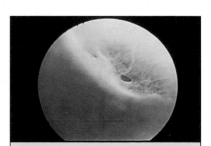

Fig. 7.81 Lattice degeneration with round hole. Courtesy of Leo Bores.

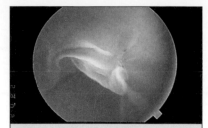

Fig. 7.82 Retinal detachment with large hole.

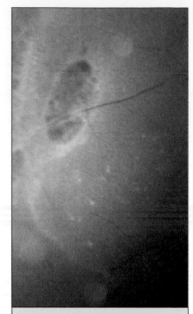

Fig. 7.83 Retinal detachment caused by large tear and hole in area of lattice degeneration.

Retinal holes and detachments (RD)

A retinal detachment is a separation of the neurosensory retina from the RPE (Fig. 7.80). Sixty-six percent of RDs begin with myopic thinning or lattice degeneration in the peripheral retina. Lattice degeneration is seen with an indirect ophthalmoscope in 8% of eyes as a white meshwork of lines with black pigment near the ora serrata (Figs 7.81 and 7.83). Holes may develop in these areas spontaneously or from trauma, cataract surgery, vitreous traction, or contraction of diabetic retinal membranes. Fluid enters the holes and detaches the retina (Figs 7.82 and 7.83). This is called a rhegmatogenous retinal detachment. Not all holes cause problems. Small, round, asymptomatic holes may often be left untreated. Large horseshoe tears with vitreous traction and recent symptoms must be sealed. Less frequently occurring is a non-rhegmatogenous RD with no holes. These may be due to choroidal effusions into the retina as occurs with choroidal tumors and scleritis. Symptoms of RD often include loss of vision, described as a "curtain", with flashes and floaters. Ophthalmoscopically, an elevated, gray membrane is seen unless a vitreous hemorrhage obscures it. Fine, reddish vitreous debris ("tobacco dust") liberated by the retina pigment epithelium may be seen with a slit lamp and should alert one to a possible retinal hole or detachment.

Surgical repair of the hole using laser, cryo, or diathermy creates a chorioretinal adhesive–scar (Fig. 7.84). Depending on the type and

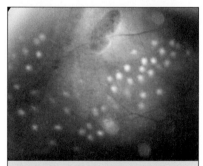

Fig. 7.84 After cryotherapy, the retinal detachment in the figure above is treated with the expansile gas C_3F_8, and positioning of the body so that the bubble tamponades the tear. Courtesy of Jiuhn-Feng Hwang, MD, San-Ni Chen. Reprinted from *Amer. J. Ophth.*, Feb. 2007, Vol. 143, No. 2, p. 217–221. Treatment of Rhegmatogenous Retinal Detachment by Pneumatic Retinopexy. With permission from Elsevier.

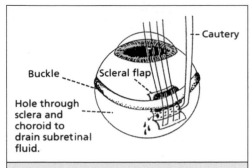

Fig. 7.85 Surgical repair of retinal detachment.

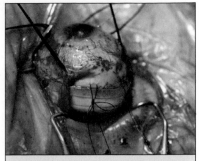

Fig. 7.86 Repair of retinal detachment with silicone scleral buckle (↑). Courtesy of Stuart Green, MD.

size of the detachment, increasingly, more complex surgery may be done. Small holes and detachments, especially at the 12 o'clock position, can be repaired with pneumatic retinopexy where a gas is injected into the vitreous. It presses the retina against the choroid and tamponades the hole by manipulating the patient's head position. Air is often used and absorbs in several days. The expansive gas perfluropropate (S_3F_8), when needed, lasts for weeks. Silicone oil is used in more complicated cases and is removed in 2–3 months. A pars plana vitrectomy is done if vitreous traction is suspected. An encircling scleral buckle (Figs 7.85 and 7.86), which pushes the sclera against the retina, may be added. In this case, subretinal fluid is drained through a scleral incision and cryo- or diathermy is applied to the retina through the sclera.

Holes in the macula (Fig. 7.87) do not usually lead to detachments, but if they are full thickness, central vision could drop to 20/400. An internal limiting membranectomy and pars plana vitrectomy could be performed if the hole is due to vitreoretinal traction bands Figs 7.87–7.89). Air is then injected into the vitreous and the patient is sent home to lie on their stomach for two weeks so that the air rises and tamponades the hole.

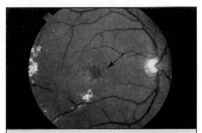

Fig. 7.87 Diabetic retinopathy with exudates and macular hole (↑).

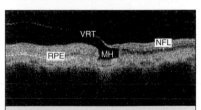

Fig. 7.88 Oct scan of macular hole caused by vitreous traction. RPE - retina pigment epithelium, NFL - nerve fiber layer, MH - macular hole, VRT - vitreoretinal traction.

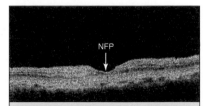

Fig. 7.89 Oct scan of macular hole resolution after vitrectomy with injection of gas into the vitreous. NFP - normal foveal pit.

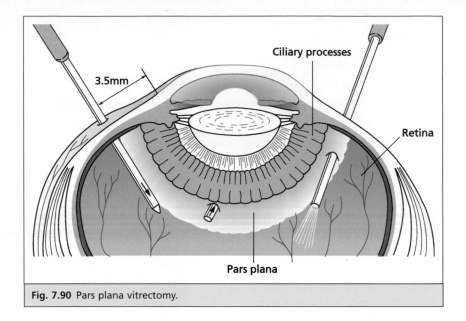

Fig. 7.90 Pars plana vitrectomy.

Pars plana vitrectomy

(Figs 7.90 and 7.91)

Vitreous surgery is performed by inserting three instruments into the eye through the anterior pars plana. This location avoids the highly vascular ciliary processes, and the delicate retina. The entry sites are located on the sclera by measuring 3.5 mm posterior to the limbus. One site is for endoillumination. The second is for irrigation with balanced saline to replace any vitreous removed. The third is for instruments which can cut and remove vitreous membranes; obtain tissue for cytology or culture; inject medications, gas, or silicone oil; cauterize or laser photocoagulate the retina; and forceps and magnets to remove foreign bodies. These procedures are performed while looking through a microscope with a contact lens on the cornea. Cataracts are a common complication followed by retinal hemorrhages, holes and detachments.

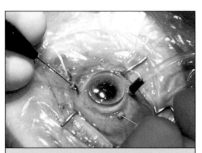

Fig. 7.91 Pars plana vitrectomy showing sites for illumination, irrigation, and aspiration. The interior of the eye is viewed using a corneal contact lens together with the operating microscope.
Courtesy of Stuart Green, MD.

Index

Manual for Eye Examination and Diagnosis, Eighth edition. Mark Leitman.
© 2012 John Wiley & Sons, Ltd. Published 2012 by John Wiley & Sons, Ltd.

Appendix 1
Hyperlipidemia

Normal blood lipids	
Normal cholesterol	<199 mg/dl
HDL cholesterol	>39 mg/dl
LDL cholesterol	<99 mg/dl
LDL/HDL	<3.6
Triglycerides	<150 mg/dl

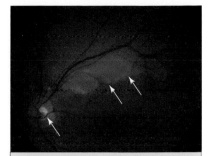

Fig. A1.1 Branch retinal artery embolus (↑) from carotid artery and resulting pale ischemic retina (↑↑). Courtesy of Elliot Davidoff, MD

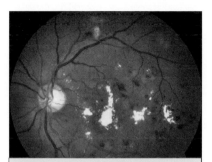

Fig. A1.2 In diabetes, hard exudates are caused by lipoproteins leaking from retinal capillaries into the extracellular space. Lowering blood fat levels help minimize this complication. Courtesy of Joanna Gosztyla.

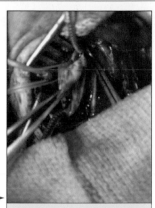

Fig. A1.4 Thrombectomy using spatula and forceps (Fig. 3.59).

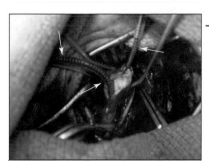

Fig. A1.3 Carotid endarterectomy showing temporary shunt (↑) to bypass surgical site. It is the gold standard for treating carotid stenosis. If contraindicated, stenting is considered. Courtesy of Niranjan Rao, MD, Chief of Vascular Surgery, St. Peter's Univ. Hospital New Brunswick, NJ.

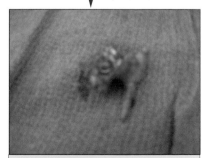

Fig. A1.5 Plaque removed from carotid artery.

Manual for Eye Examination and Diagnosis, Eighth edition. Mark Leitman.
© 2012 John Wiley & Sons, Ltd. Published 2012 by John Wiley & Sons, Ltd.

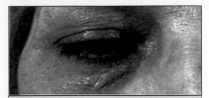

Fig. A1.6 Xanthelasma are irregular, yellowish plaques on the medial side of the upper and lower lids. They are often inherited and sometimes associated with hypercholesterolemia and a 51% increased risk of heart attack.

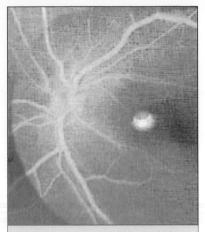

Fig. A1.7 Creamy, white retinal blood vessels indicating lipemia retinalis which occurs with triglyceride levels >2,500 mg/dl. This patient had triglycerides 29,000 mg/dl and cholesterol 1,470. Courtesy of Murat Ozdemir, MD and *Ophthal. Surg. Laser Imaging* 2003; 34:221–22.

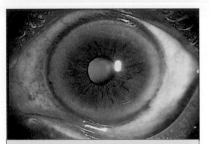

Fig. A1.8 Corneal arcus is a narrow, white band of lipid infiltration separated from the limbus by a clear zone. It occurs in everyone by age 80. Its occurence in those younger than 50 warrants measuring blood lipids, which may be elevated.

Appendix 2
Amsler grid

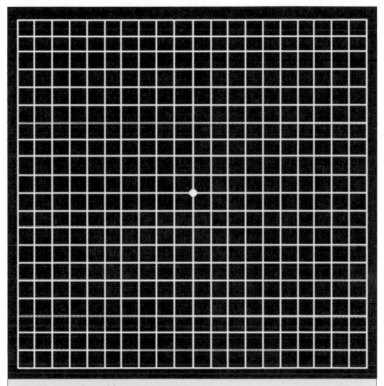

Fig. A2.1 Amsler grid.

1. Wear best corrected lenses for near.
2. Hold card at 14 inches.
3. Cover one eye.
4. Focus on central dot.
5. Detect any wavy, distorted or blind areas.

Manual for Eye Examination and Diagnosis, Eighth edition. Mark Leitman.
© 2012 John Wiley & Sons, Ltd. Published 2012 by John Wiley & Sons, Ltd.

Appendix

Amlet and